W9-BLN-020

NORTH COUNTRY LIBRARY SYSTEM
Watertown, New York

WOMEN AND ALOPECIA

Managing Unexplained Hair Loss

CENTRAL LIBRARY
WATERTOWN

L. Lee Culvert

YOUR HEALTH PRESS

Women and Alopecia: Managing Unexplained Hair Loss
First published by Your Health Press in association with Trafford Publishing.

Cover and Text Design: www.729design.com
Cover Photo: www.iStockphoto.com

Important Notice:
The purpose of this book is to educate. It is sold with the understanding that the author and publisher shall have neither liability nor responsibility for any injury caused or alleged to be caused directly or indirectly by the information contained in this book. While every effort has been made to ensure its accuracy, the book's contents should not be construed as medical advice. Each person's health needs are unique. To obtain recommendations appropriate to your particular situation, please consult a qualified health care provider.

All trademarked products appear herein minus the registered trademark symbol.

©Copyright 2009 L. Lee Culvert and Your Health Press
All rights reserved. No part of this publication may be reproduced, stored in a retrieval system, or transmitted, in any form or by any means, electronic, mechanical, photocopying, recording, or otherwise, without the written prior permission of the author.

Note for Librarians: A cataloguing record for this book is available from Library and Archives Canada at www.collectionscanada.ca/amicus/index-e.html
isbn: 978-1-4269-0014-3

Printed in Victoria, BC, Canada.

Order this book online at www.trafford.com
or email orders@trafford.com

Most Trafford titles are also available at major online book retailers. We at Trafford believe that it is the responsibility of us all, as both individuals and corporations, to make choices that are environmentally and socially sound. You, in turn, are supporting this responsible conduct each time you purchase a Trafford book, or make use of our publishing services. To find out how you are helping, please visit www.trafford.com/responsiblepublishing.html.

Our mission is to efficiently provide the world's finest, most comprehensive book publishing service, enabling every author to experience success. To find out how to publish your book, your way, and have it available worldwide, visit us online at www.trafford.com/10510.

www.trafford.com
North America & international
toll-free: 1 888 232 4444 (USA & Canada)
phone: 250 383 6864 fax: 250 383 6804 email: info@trafford.com
Th e United Kingdom & Europe
phone: +44 (0)1865 487 395 local rate: 0845 230 9601
facsimile: +44 (0)1865 481 507 email: info.uk@trafford.com

WOMEN AND ALOPECIA

Managing Unexplained Hair Loss

OTHER *YOUR HEALTH PRESS* TITLES

Stopping Cancer at the Source: The Primary Prevention of Cancer, 2nd edition by M. Sara Rosenthal, Ph.D. (2008)

The PCOS Diet Cookbook: Delicious Recipes and Tips for Women with PCOS on the Low GI Diet by Nadir R. Farid, M.D. and Norene Gilletz (2007)

Coping with Molar Pregnancy and Choriocarcinoma by Tara Johnson and Meredith Schwartz (2007)

Preventing Menopause: How to Stop Menopause Before It Starts by Beth Rosenshein (2006)

Living Well with Celiac Disease: Abundance Beyond Wheat and Gluten, 2nd edition by Claudine Crangle (2006)

The Low-Iodine Diet Cookbook: Easy and Delicious Recipes and Tips for Thyroid Cancer Patients by Norene Gilletz (2005)

Menopause Before 40: Coping with Premature Ovarian Failure by Karin Banerd (2004)

Healing Injuries the Natural Way: How to Mend Bones, Muscles, Tendons & More by Michelle Cook (2004)

Thyroid Eye Disease: Understanding Graves' Ophthalmopathy by Elaine A. Moore (2003)

Living Well with an Ostomy by Elizabeth Rayson (2003)

The Thyroid Cancer Book, 2nd edition by M. Sara Rosenthal, Ph.D. (2003)

TABLE OF CONTENTS

INTRODUCTION: WHY A BOOK ON HAIR LOSS IN WOMEN

It started as a personal matter. Blessed with a good head of baby-fine hair that I wore straight and shoulder-length from childhood into college, and then through most of my adult life, I first noticed in my early fifties that I was having bad hair days more often, and then that I was becoming a flat head. I couldn't get my hair to appear full no matter where I parted it or how much I had it trimmed or what shampoo or conditioner I used. What was going on here? Red-faced, I confided in my hair stylist and she agreed— my hair was thinner than it had been just months before. We could "fix it" she offered, by cutting it to chin length and layering. "Go ahead," was all I could offer in return, and watched while she proceeded to trim and layer the all-one-length bob I'd worn for years, turning it into a shorter, and I have to admit, more flattering, more angular version that I've grown to like. It not only made my hair look thicker as my hairdresser had promised, it was more interesting and livelier, making me feel livelier, too. At that time, I didn't tell her that I was taking an immunosuppressant for rheumatoid arthritis, because it simply didn't occur to me that this drug could be a cause of thinning hair. I also didn't discuss my age and the inevitable thinning associated with aging, because I didn't know it happened to nearly every middle-aged woman. Too many things were expected to happen in middle age and, quite simply, I didn't want to go there. And, like most women who notice hair loss or thinning, I suffered in silence; I didn't consult a physician or even mention it to my rheumatologist. Men went bald. Women didn't. I was not going bald.

No matter how closely I examined the counter around my bathroom sink or the shower drain or my hairbrush, I honestly didn't see any signs of excess hair actually falling out of my scalp. I more or less (and reluctantly) concluded that this whole thinning hair thing had to be just another facet of aging—one more aspect of middle age that I'd have to get used to. However, I was a professional medical writer and, for me, literature searches were the norm, so I dug into my medical texts and online resources and, sure enough, the drug I was taking showed up as a possible cause of hair loss. It was low on the list of possible causes of drug-induced hair loss, but it was there nevertheless. I also learned that androgenetic alopecia was the most common form of hair loss and that it affected all men and nearly all women to some degree. Imagine! The more I looked, the more I found. And I was amazed at the number of hair loss conditions that affected women, especially when I had lived to middle age thinking that only men had receding hairlines or became bald. I also learned fairly quickly that this idea prevailed in our society. In reading further and talking to women and physicians, I learned that all medical practices deal with hair loss or diseases that can cause it, that hundreds of conditions and a handful of drugs can lead to hair loss, and that clinical research on hair loss is lacking, primarily because it's not a life-threatening condition like cancer or heart disease. The personal matter fast became a project at that point and this book is the culmination. I'm satisfied that I've researched a topic that has been sadly neglected in communications to the public—even with the devastating psychological effects that losing hair can produce. Women now have a comprehensive discussion of the many forms of hair loss and a range of medical and cosmetic options for addressing them.

EXPLAINING UNEXPLAINED HAIR LOSS

Hair loss, referred to clinically as alopecia, affects both women and men across all age groups—and the most common type of hair loss, even though it has been called "male pattern baldness," affects millions of women as well as millions of men. Assuming that you have acquired this book because you or someone close to you has noticed some degree of hair loss, the first thing you need to know is how common hair loss is among our population—and among women.

Gender differences related to hair loss are primarily in the numbers of people affected. In the United States alone, 21 million women have noticeable hair loss of the "male pattern baldness" type, described clinically as androgenetic alopecia, and these days described more accurately as simply "pattern baldness." This common type of baldness also affects 35 million men in the United States. Approximately 40 percent of women in the United States experience hair loss of some kind at some point during their life, not just through androgenetic alopecia alone, but from all types of alopecia. Meanwhile, 35 percent of men in the United States experience hair loss by age 35; and among men aged 60 and older, the rate increases to 65 percent. Again, this is primarily male pattern baldness, but these statistics also include other types of hair loss. I will be addressing all of them in our comprehensive hair loss story.

Women and Alopecia

Hair loss is experienced universally and affects people of different genders, ages, races, and nationalities around the globe, vastly multiplying hair loss statistics worldwide when compared to U.S. hair loss statistics alone. Although few distinctions exist among members of the human species—that is, we all share the same bone structure, muscular structure, basic body chemistry, and cellular makeup—hair characteristics can differentiate us. Hair follicles on different heads produce hairs that vary in color, shape, thickness, length, and strength. Although the tendency to lose hair is relatively the same among races and nationalities, the way in which hair loss occurs can be an area of difference. The incidence of androgenetic alopecia (AGA), for example, which is the pattern hair loss that is believed to affect nearly all people to some degree, varies among ethnic groups. Among men in early adulthood, the incidence of AGA in black and Asian men is only one fourth of that found in white males, and among older individuals it increases to one third of the incidence among white men. Differences also occur between genders and *within* racial groups. If we look around at the people we know and live with, we can see that even within families we have blonds, brunettes, short hair, long hair, thick hair, and … no hair.

Among individuals of Asian heritage, scalps are covered with fewer hairs per square inch, resulting in lower hair density than in most Caucasians or most people of African descent. At the same time, because the hair follicles of people of Asian descent are actually thicker, the visual appearance is that the head of hair is thicker. These characteristics make Asian women especially subject to developing hair that thins evenly around their head. This is a general characteristic, however, so it is not universal among Asian populations. Among this population, we see curly hair, light brown and reddish hair, thick and thin heads of hair … and even receding hairlines and baldness. Caucasians, too, are all over the map with hair characteristics, primarily because of various inherited familial traits stemming from mixed nationalities and races. Individuals of African heritage, on the other hand, characteristically have naturally curly hair, as do a substantial number of people of Mediterranean descent. Because my own hair is thin and straight, even though I have a lot of it, I've been jealous all my life of curly hair; it's so impressive to me with its appearance of fullness and greater hair density over the entire head. It turns out that the hair follicles of people with curly hair actually curve more than follicles on the heads of people with straight hair. Since curly-haired individuals can become bald along with everyone else, this characteristic makes hair transplants particularly difficult, since donor hairs, which are typically taken from the back of the individual's head, are from similarly curved hair follicles that are at risk of being easily severed when hair is harvested for transplant.

Perhaps the only conclusion that can be made here, despite differences in follicles and hair traits, is that we all have hair problems. And although hair loss is just one of them, it's the one we least want, and one that can be potentially difficult to diagnose and treat.

THE HAIR LOSS WE HAVE IN COMMON

All individuals are believed to have some degree of the most common form of hair loss mentioned above, androgenetic alopecia—a condition, as the name suggests, related to genetic makeup and the presence in the body of an androgen called dihydrotestosterone (DHT). Yes, that's a hormone (androgens are male hormones), and by middle age, many men and some women will have a condition in which male hormone activity causes changes in the normal hair growth cycle, eventually resulting in losing hair or thinning hair. Androgenetic hair loss is actually believed to start somewhere between the early teens and age 40, but according to studies of men and women with hair loss, it will not usually become visible until age 50 or later. The condition is more noticeable in some individuals than in others, and occurs more in men than in women, sometimes even in men in their 20s and 30s. We may see signs of thinning, balding, or receding hairlines in some people, and consider it to be fairly normal—and to some extent it is. Although androgenetic alopecia is the most common cause of hair loss in females, we are less apt to see it in women simply because hairstyling is often able to make the condition less noticeable. In this way, women's hairstyling possibilities can be a wonderful advantage, but unfortunately, alopecia has forms that cannot hide behind a hairstyle. These forms all fit somewhere under the heading of "unexplained hair loss," and my purpose in writing this book is to help explain the forms it can take, and also to explain more about the more common androgenetic hair loss.

What happens when women begin to notice thinning or receding hair? Does it happen to all women to some degree? What are the possible causes of hair loss? And why do some women begin to experience hair loss in a particular pattern of loss, such as small, quarter-size bare spots on the scalp or a part,

13

that is becoming wider and wider? These and other examples of unexplained hair loss are the topics addressed in this book. If you or someone you know has seen signs of hair loss for reasons unknown or unexplained, you may be able to find your condition described within these pages, learn how and why it may occur, how it is typically diagnosed, and what options you may have to do something about it. Hundreds of "cures" are available and cosmetic solutions as well; some are valid and others may be bogus and filled with false hope. You'll get the inside story on promising treatments and false promises. You will also learn that you are not alone—thousands of women are affected by hair loss every year—and you will learn that wigs, or staying at home in the shadows, are not the only solutions.

I have written *Women and Alopecia: Managing Unexplained Hair Loss* using reliable information from medical texts, clinical research reports, trusted Web sites, and patient information provided by practitioners who have treated hair loss. Besides describing in detail the most common hair loss disorders that affect women—along with a few that are not so common—I provide discussions of the way your hair grows normally; what can change the cycle of your hair growth; the importance of early and accurate diagnosis; and what medical, surgical, and cosmetic treatment options are available. Chapter 8 discusses caring for and maintaining healthy hair. I even touch on the images of hair we hold in our mind, the ingrained ideas that make having a head of hair so important culturally. In fact, I begin with this last topic and try to answer the question of why hair loss can be such a devastating experience, especially for women.

As a postscript, I'm happy to say that my thinning hair has never become any thinner; the condition was either not progressive or it possibly reversed on its own when my dosage of immunosuppressant was reduced. Because I was not diagnosed, I still don't really know whether I'm one of the 21 million or so women who have genetically induced female pattern hair loss or whether the drug I was taking caused my temporary thinning. I haven't gone back to the old hairstyle. I'm still enjoying the new one, but for the record, *I have* continued to use rosemary volumizing hair shampoo and conditioner—I'm middle aged, after all, and my research found that we're all in line for thinner hair at some point. Meanwhile, I'm hoping that *your* hair loss condition, whatever it is, will be as correctable and short lived as mine was. But, with all that I've learned, I urge you not to do as I did—don't put your head in the sand and just hope your hair loss problem goes away. Women *do* lose hair and today we have access to accurate diagnosis and good options for treating it, either medically, surgically or cosmetically. By all means, see a dermatologist and find out what's up with your hair.

CHAPTER 1

THE IMPORTANCE OF HAIR: HOW WE FEEL ABOUT IT, WHAT CAN HAPPEN TO IT

How we feel about hair and hair loss, what alopecia is, what forms it takes, what forms affect women, difference between alopecia and hair loss from chemotherapy, scarring and nonscarring forms of alopecia, who gets alopecia, common perceptions about women and hair loss, who treats hair loss

THE ROMANCE OF HAIR

"Rapunzel, Rapunzel, let down your hair." Remember this familiar request by the fairy-tale heroine's significant other? He stands at the foot of the tower where Rapunzel is being held against her will and begs that she let down her long, long hair so that he can climb up this mane and rescue her. Remember, too, the biblical story of Sampson, whose hair was believed to be the source of his strength? He lost that strength dramatically when his wife, Delilah, cut his hair as he slept. Surely she must have believed, as his enemies did, that he had "the power" as long as he had his hair.

In Rapunzel's story, her beauty—specifically the beauty of her hair—was clearly identified as the key to her desirability, and maybe the way in which she influenced her partner's behavior as well. In Sampson's story, the loss of hair is symbolically associated with loss of power—perhaps even loss of virility. These fictionalized, romanticized versions of qualities associated with having a full and beautiful head of hair may not be so different from ideas held about hair at various times in history and among different populations around the world. To Buddhist or early Christian monks, for example, shaving the head was considered to be a sign of renouncing worldly attachments. Shaved heads clearly identified slaves among the general populace in ancient Greek and Roman cultures. In Western culture, even into modern times, military recruits are treated to a severe haircut as soon as they enter the service. Military officers, and sometimes military policies, have even used the shaving of soldiers' heads as a way to dehumanize, and thereby control, their own soldiers and to punish captured enemy soldiers—in both cases letting the shaved ones know who was boss. In the 1960s, ironically, the young men who grew their hair long or tied it in a ponytail were considered by some to be weaker and more sissified than more conservative short-haired men. We didn't all agree on this, of course. More recently, the bald heads of skinheads have been seen as symbols of aggression, and the shaved heads of some women have been interpreted as a protest against traditional male-pleasing gestures or, perhaps, more accurately to the women themselves, a symbol of being in control of their own life. Irish singer Sinead O'Connor, for example, made a strong public statement with her baldness. And when a young American pop star tried to do the same, Dr. Linda Blair, a California-based clinical psychologist, explained to reporters that the shaved head of a woman is seen by the public as shocking or a sign of personal crisis because flowing hair is linked to the notion of feminine beauty and reproduction.

Can it be true—do we really manipulate opinion with our hairstyles? Where do we stand on this idea that our hair says something about us? And how do today's associations with hair compare to those in fairy tales and historical images?

Hair has been referred to as our "crowning glory." You can probably think of dozens of other words and phrases you may have heard or read that describe hair as beautiful, shiny, thick, sleek, slicked back, a lion's mane, fair-haired, big hair, curly locks, hair that "cascades down her back," and so on. Goldilocks is the heroine of a popular children's book and she has a fairly clear association with purity and innocence. Even the notion that "blondes have more fun" suggests a personality trait associated with hair color. And the familiar line "silver threads among the gold" romances aging hair. We can find phrases and images in literature, theater, television, movies, and opera that suggest the allure and power of hair. With these images held subliminally in our cultural mind-set, it may not be surprising that the psychosocial response to losing hair includes fear and a loss of self-image or self-worth. Hair today and through the ages has been a symbol of attractiveness, sex appeal and sexual prowess, mental powers, and physical superiority. There seems to be no end to public reactions and comments on extreme hairstyles and what they might suggest. However, private reactions are generally kept private, especially where hair loss or balding is concerned, and this, too, says something about the effects of hair problems. What do we think it says about us if we *lose* our hair?

WHY WE HATE LOSING HAIR

Hair loss is not deadly; it will not shorten our life or kill us. Why, then, does the prospect of losing hair provoke panic in otherwise strong, stable individuals and cause embarrassment, shame, and depression in men and women who have developed a receding hairline, bare patches, hair thinning, or baldness? The very thought of hair loss seems to raise all kinds of personal feelings, emotions, expectations, and fears. We can't explain precisely why it's a troublesome topic, but after reviewing patients reactions to hair loss, I concluded we all share a deep fear of losing our hair. When we lose hair, perhaps we feel we're losing some part of our deeper selves with it.

As humans, male or female, we become quite used to our facial features and usually accept them, whatever they might be. There seems to be little choice but to accept. Or perhaps we could rationalize: A big nose? Well, it's just like my dad's nose and it looks fine on him. A crooked smile? Hey, nobody else smiles like me; it makes me unique. On the other hand, our hair never seems to make us happy. We change it constantly and suffer "bad hair days" when we "can't do anything with it." At some level, we know our hair may suffer when we suffer an illness, and will likely change as we age, even though we can't exactly predict specific changes. We women may look at our bald dads and think, "Thank goodness I'm female." Meanwhile, we cut our hair, let it grow, color it, bleach it, curl it, and straighten it at will. We're apt to change our hairstyle at the drop of a hat. Whether we choose straight styles, curls, dreads, ponytails, up-sweeps, twists, Afros, special weaves, or shocking Day-Glo colors, we're saying something about how we'd like to present ourselves at any given time. Sure, our motivation to alter our outward appearance could be to reinvent what the world sees, or it could possibly be connected with a need or desire to alter the images we hold of ourselves. Could self-image, after all, be at the root of our reaction to hair loss?

STRESS—A CAUSE AND A SYMPTOM OF HAIR LOSS

Clinical studies of men and women with hair loss find that individuals with alopecia commonly experience loss of self-image right along with loss of hair. Although physicians consider hair loss to be a benign medical condition— one that doesn't threaten patients' lives or result in progressive or severe illness—they report that the emotions of patients who are losing hair can sometimes skyrocket out of proportion to the extent of the underlying hair problem. This may be the physicians' perspective, but it's not necessarily the perspective of patients, to whom all degrees of hair loss conjure up pictures of baldness. It's not hard to understand why strong emotions are a common response, and research bears it out. Emotional or psychological disturbances that come with hair loss have been shown in studies to interfere with or reduce a patient's overall sense of well-being. Studies have also shown that hair loss is disturbing to both sexes, but study conclusions repeatedly report that women are more profoundly affected than men. Whether or not the hair loss can be corrected, the stigma attached to hair loss among women has proven to be extremely stressful. Women report feeling too embarrassed to purchase a medicine or cosmetic product, when they finally decide to try one, then they report feeling frustrated with the less-than-satisfying results of using these products. Consequently, women are more likely to explore extreme methods of correction for their problem, desperately seeking experimental treatments and creative cosmetic methods to conceal hair loss. The psychological effects may continue even while treatment is being sought or temporary cover-ups are being used. Hair loss hurts—the emotional aspects need to be addressed along with the clinical.

Fortunately, as knowledge and experience increase in the hair loss realm, the range of emotions and reactions that develop as a response to hair loss are beginning to be considered actual symptoms—symptoms just as significant as physical symptoms. And, along with advances in treating hair loss and surgical replacement of scalp hair, psychological treatment is becoming a standard part of medical treatment. Your doctor may be able to recommend local sources of help and support, and hair loss organizations across the country have resources in place if you need them (see Resources).

Meanwhile, somewhere short of having a recognized hair loss condition, we're all losing hair all the time—and it's quite natural. Let's take a look at how much hair loss constitutes a hair loss problem.

NATURAL SHEDDING OF HAIR

We all shed hair, some more, some less. We see hair in sink and tub drains, on our shoulders, and in our combs and brushes. If we're really paying attention, we may notice that more hair is shed in fall and winter than in spring or summer. This is not an accident; it's a direct result, not of temperature, but of sunlight. It turns out that hormones are particularly sensitive to changes in exposure to daylight. In fact, when mink and other mammals have been studied, levels of a protein hormone involved in the secretion of milk (prolactin) have been shown to be significantly altered. Prolactin is a hormone that triggers molting in animals. It's not a surprise, then, that human mammals have a similar molting process. We just need to remember that this normal shedding is temporary and actual hair loss is not taking place, because shed hairs are usually being replaced through the normal hair growth cycle as quickly as they are being shed. We don't need Rogaine to correct normal shedding of this type, we may only need a change of season. (Note: Rogaine is a registered trademark of McNeil Laboratories.)

COMMON HAIR LOSS DISORDERS: ARE THEY ALL "ALOPECIA"?

Alopecia is a medical term used to describe hair loss—hair loss of any kind, on any part of the body, although the loss of scalp hair is most common and most disturbing. Alopecia refers specifically to abnormal conditions that cause hair to fall out and conditions that prevent or discourage hair from growing in normal cycles. But even if hair is lost because of behavioral causes or parasites, the resulting hair loss is still called alopecia.

All forms of alopecia can be described generally under two types of disorders:

1. Disorders that involve normal hair follicles and abnormal cycles of hair growth
2. Disorders that originate from damaged hair follicles

You can see, then, that alopecia is a disorder, not of the hair itself, but of the skin of the scalp and other body skin surfaces on which hair grows. Wherever hair grows on the body, the skin surface will have hair follicles through which individual hairs grow. Any processes, conditions, or illnesses that affect the health of hair follicles may cause hair loss or changes in hair growth. The cycle of hair growth, for example, involves periods of hair follicle activity (anagen phase) and periods of rest (telogen phase). When either of these cycles is altered by any cause, some degree of hair loss—or alopecia—is a possible result.

Hair loss can occur on the scalp, ranging from small bare patches to larger or more diffuse areas of loss, sometimes following definitive patterns. In some types of alopecia, hair loss may occur on other parts of the body, including arms, legs, and pubic region, and also, in men, facial hair, chest hair, and back hair. Some forms of alopecia are directly or indirectly related to traumatic events or periods of stress. This type of alopecia may also reveal previously unidentified androgenetic alopecia, the pattern type of hair loss (male pattern baldness) that is related to male hormones and aging, even if it occurs in women. However, if no androgenetic alopecia is found, the hair loss condition caused by trauma may reverse within two to three months after the causative event. Certain drugs are known to cause hair loss, to stimulate hair growth, or to cause changes in the shape and color of hair. Types and amount of hair loss usually depend on the way the drug works in the body, the drug dosage, and the susceptibility of the individuals taking the drug. Damage to follicles or hair loss itself may be reversible if the drug is discontinued. Although many drugs occasionally cause some hair loss, only a few have been proven to affect hair growth, usually by increasing the period of rest in the growth cycle, but some also increase the period of growth. A somewhat controversial cause of hair loss involves iron deficiency; experts disagree on the possible role of iron in hair loss and even disagree on what precisely constitutes iron deficiency—either reduced levels of iron-bearing hemoglobin in the blood or reduced levels of serum ferritin, a marker for iron content in the blood. Another group of alopecias are called *effluviums*, affecting either the rest phase of hair growth (telogen effluvium) or the growing phase (anagen effluvium) or both. Telogen effluvium occurs when the number of hair follicles not growing hair during a rest phase increases, or said the opposite way, when decreases occur in the number of hair follicles in the growth phase. This situation, fortunately, can usually be reversed. Meanwhile, we have to be mindful of the fact that not all types of alopecia have that expected outcome.

Generally speaking, forms of hair loss other than androgenetic alopecia will occur in very few individuals in the whole population. The nonandrogenetic forms seen most often are telogen effluvium, alopecia areata, and cicatricial or "scarring" alopecia. Practicing dermatologists may see only a few of these forms of hair loss in all the years of their practice, and this lack of experience may not be helpful to the person who has a rare form of alopecia—another clue to the inherent difficulty in diagnosing hair loss conditions.

Just to familiarize you with alopecia in general, I will now summarize the most prevalent types of alopecia; however, you can find a more detailed discussion of each type in chapter 3, which discusses the signs, symptoms, and causes of alopecia.

COMMON FORMS OF ALOPECIA

Common hair loss disorders or forms of alopecia are described here briefly under two general categories: alopecia with normal hair follicles and abnormal hair growth, and alopecia that stems from damaged hair follicles. A third category refers to hair loss that occurs as a result of certain behavior. All of the forms described here are discussed in more detail in the chapters that follow.

Forms of Alopecia with Normal Hair Follicles and Abnormal Hair Growth

Androgenetic alopecia—the most common form of hair loss, often referred to as "male pattern baldness," and related to the presence of the male hormone dihydrotestosterone (DHT). Androgenetic alopecia, as the name implies, is considered to be hereditary, or related to certain genes inherited from family members. It is believed to affect all individuals, male and female, to some degree and at various age levels, although it may never become noticeable. If it does become noticed, it will not be until the individual is in his or her fifties or later. (See "Androgenetic Alopecia," chapter 3.)

Alopecia areata—patchy hair loss, hair falling out as a result of an auto-immune process. It typically begins with a single oval patch or a group of patches of well-defined bare areas; this form of alopecia can remain confined to a few bare patches or can eventually involve balding of the entire head. (See "Alopecia Areata," chapter 3.)

Telogen effluvium—diffuse hair loss that occurs when normal phases of growth and rest are disrupted, resulting in an abnormally long or out-of-sync rest phase; it is sometimes called *traumatic alopecia* because the shifts in growth and rest phases can follow a traumatic event, severe stress, or use of certain medications. Iron deficiency and thyroid disease are just two of a range of possible causes. Iron deficiency can cause hair loss in otherwise healthy people, primarily women of child-bearing age. This sometimes unexplained hair loss may be associated with reduced levels of serum ferritin, a measure of iron in the blood, or reduced hemoglobin, the iron-bearing protein in the blood. Ferritin supplementation may help to correct low hemoglobin and hair loss. Hair loss associated with iron deficiency is a form of telogen effluvium. Hair loss is common in individuals with untreated hypothyroidism (low thyroid hormone). In cases of hypothyroidism, hair loss is a form of telogen effluvium, and is corrected when thyroid hormone levels are restored. In cases of hyperthyroidism (when the thyroid gland is overactive) or in cases of thyrotoxicosis (when there is too much thyroid hormone circulating in the body), which is frequently caused by taking too high a dosage of thyroid hormone to correct hypothyroidism, upsetting hair changes may also occur. Both hyperthyroidism and thyrotoxicosis can cause transient changes in the nature of hair—the hair shafts are finer, but there is not typically thinning of the hair on the scalp. Beta blockers, which are prescribed for hyperthyroidism or thyrotoxicosis, are a class of drugs that can cause telogen effluvium, but no other drugs used to treat thyroid disease cause hair loss. It's important to note that anyone being treated for thyroid disease could experience hormonal fluctuations due to the nature of thyroid disease, and hair loss could result if hypothyroidism is not treated. According to numerous sources, there is an association of hair loss with a range of thyroid medications or thyroid conditions. It's also important to note that thyroid disease is often an autoimmune disease. Autoimmune diseases tend to cluster; so if you have an autoimmune thyroid disease, you may be more at risk for autoimmune alopecia. (See "Telogen Effluvium," chapter 3.)

Forms of Alopecia with Damaged Hair Follicles

Alopecia universalis—hair loss or absence of hair on entire scalp and body—even eyebrows and eyelashes are missing and no facial hair grows. It is usually apparent from the time of birth and is associated with genetic causes. (See "Alopecia Universalis," chapter 3.)

Cicatricial alopecia—a scarring form of hair loss that occurs because of damage to the underlying scalp and to hair follicles; the scalp itself will appear abnormal, having been damaged by infections such as syphilis, tuberculosis, acquired immunodeficiency syndrome (AIDS), or herpes. It can also be the result of autoimmune disease, injuries, burns, or radiation therapy. (See "Cicatricial Alopecia," chapter 3.)

Traction alopecia (also called traumatic alopecia, or cosmetic alopecia)—hair loss caused by grooming styles that create high tension and breakage of hairs, and by repetitive hairstyling practices that damage hair follicles. Tight braiding and ponytails (e.g., cornrows or dreadlocks), use of curling irons, brush rollers, chemical treatments (e.g., perms, straightening agents, coloring, or bleaching products), or hairbrushes with square or angled tips have also been known to cause traumatic alopecia. (See "Traction Alopecia," chapter 3.)

Tinea capitis—a fungal infection that affects the scalp; it usually occurs in young people between age ten and early teens, and hair loss can be reversed if scarring is minimal. (See "Tinea Capitis," chapter 3.)

Other Forms of Alopecia

Trichotillomania—a form of hair loss that starts with a behavior problem and, unlike other forms of alopecia, does not involve hair follicles. Instead, "trich" is the compulsive pulling and plucking of one's own hair—scalp hair, eyelashes and eyebrows, hair on the forearms or pubic hair—a behavioral characteristic usually associated with a traumatic life event or ongoing stress of some kind. Psychologists consider trichotillomania to be an impulse disorder rather than a compulsion. This form of hair loss is usually reversible with effective behavior modification or psychotherapy that addresses the underlying psychological causes. (See "Trichotillomania," chapter 3.)

Postoperative hair loss—occurs after cosmetic surgery, namely the brow lift, in which hair is lost in scarring just above the forehead behind the frontal hairline. Scars may be unsightly and considerably whiter or lighter than the surrounding scalp. Hair transplantation usually has good results with losses of this type.

Drug-induced hair loss—hair loss can be a result of taking certain drugs, as we just described earlier in the discussion of beta blockers, a class of drugs used for treating hyperthyroidism or thyrotoxicosis. Medications can also cause unwanted hair growth or cause changes in hair color or in the shape of individual hairs. The most significant hair loss occurs as a result of the toxic effect of cytostatic or cytotoxic drugs used for chemotherapy (anagen arrest), but other drugs used in treating a wide array of symptoms and conditions are also capable of damaging the hair matrix, resulting in various degrees of shedding, thinning, or balding. In drug-induced hair loss, removal of the offending drug usually restores the normal hair growth cycle. (See "Anagen Effluvium" chapter 3.)

DIFFERENCES BETWEEN HAIR LOSS FROM CANCER TREATMENT AND OTHER FORMS OF ALOPECIA

Chemotherapy involves the use of cell-killing chemical substances (chemotherapeutic agents called cytostatic or cytotoxic drugs) that destroy or prevent the continued growth of cancerous cells. Radiation is used in this way, too, to shrink tumors and to help prevent cancer from spreading into the cells of nearby organs. Sometimes these therapies are used singly, and sometimes together, depending on the type of cancer and the patient's response to treatment. When cancer patients lose their hair while being treated with chemotherapy or local irradiation of tumors, the hair loss that follows is a result of *anagen arrest*, or *anagen effluvium*, a condition of the hair growth cycle in which follicle activity is suspended. The descriptive terms, anagen arrest and anagen effluvium, refer to an alteration that occurs in the anagen phase of hair growth when cells have been so traumatized by the chemotherapy agent or radiation treatment that they do not divide and multiply as usual to produce new growth. Instead, when this normal cell process is halted, hair shafts break below the scalp level and hairs begin to shed between two and three weeks after the cell-destroying therapy was administered. Since the anagen phase of hair growth typically involves 85 to 90 percent of scalp hairs at any given time, hair loss can occur rapidly over the complete scalp. However, anagen arrest is a nonscarring form of hair loss that does not permanently alter hair follicles, and as soon as chemotherapy or radiation treatments stop, follicle activity and hair growth will begin again. Anagen effluvium (also called toxic alopecia) is described in chapter 3, including chemical insults or drug-related causes other than chemotherapy or radiation.

DIFFERENCES BETWEEN SCARRING AND NONSCARRING FORMS OF ALOPECIA

The different types of alopecia you've just read about can also be described as *scarring* or *nonscarring*, which has a lot to do with the potential for reversing the hair loss problem. Scarring forms of alopecia result in damage to hair follicles—possibly permanent damage—and physical examination of the scalp by the naked eye will show individual follicles or "follicular units," often surrounded by redness (erythema), scaling, or inflammation. Nonscarring forms of alopecia do not involve damage to follicles and follicular units cannot be seen when the scalp is examined. In fact, the scalp may look perfectly normal.

25

- *Scarring alopecia*—includes cicatricial alopecia, folliculitis, hair loss associated with lupus erythematosus, chronic trichotillomania, or traction alopecia, and fungus infections such as lichen planopilaris
- *Nonscarring alopecia*—includes androgenetic alopecia, telogen effluvium regardless of cause, alopecia areata, acute trichotillomania, drug-induced anagen effluvium, and syphilitic alopecia related to venereal disease

WHO ARE WE TALKING ABOUT WHEN WE TALK ABOUT HAIR LOSS?

The demographics of hair loss—that is, who among both genders and all age groups are most likely to be at risk for hair loss—differ among the various types of alopecia.

Our best chances of losing hair are related, first of all, to traits we have inherited from the families of either of our parents. We have already learned that the most common form of hair loss, androgenetic alopecia, refers to hair loss occurring in men and women as a result of genetics and the presence of the androgen dihydrotestosterone (DHT). Fifty percent of all individuals have visible hair loss by the time they are 50 years old as a result of genetically induced androgenetic alopecia. In men, this type of hair loss starts as early as age 12 and can become noticeable at any age, but is most typically seen by age 50. Women, too, may experience hair loss between their 20s and middle age, but more typically, losses usually don't usually start before age 50 and may never become noticeable. According to the International Society of Hair Restoration Surgery, female pattern alopecia (female AGA) has been estimated to occur in about 20 percent of all women in the United States, including 3 percent of women in their 20s, 17 percent of women between ages 30 and 50, and 25 to 28 percent of women over age 50. Some discussions of hair loss, however, suggest that many cases of androgenetic hair loss go unreported because only the woman herself sees the loss, and she will most likely accept it while learning to mask minor losses with smart hairstyles. However, not all evidence agrees with this theory. A study published in *Dermatologic Surgery* (Norwood, 2001), for example, suggests that the incidence of female androgenetic alopecia is actually increasing. Dr. Norwood's study showed that the increased incidence of female AGA represents hair loss occurring during and after menopause. It is also seems possible that the "increased incidence" could be a result of increased recognition and acceptance of women's hair loss as a medical problem, which could definitely encourage more women to report their hair loss conditions and seek medical help.

Autoimmune alopecia, the form called alopecia areata, occurs in 1 to 2 percent of the population, affecting men and women equally and children and young adults more often than older adults. About 60 percent of individuals treated for alopecia areata developed their first patchy hair loss before age twenty. It is the third most common type of hair loss following androgenetic alopecia and telogen effluvium. The risk for autoimmune alopecia areata is higher (37 percent) among individuals whose family history includes other autoimmune diseases such as rheumatoid arthritis, lupus, diabetes mellitus, or thyroid disease. The National Alopecia Areata Foundation (see Resources) reports that nearly 4.5 million people will develop alopecia areata within their lifetime.

Hair loss due to telogen effluvium, we have learned, comes from any condition or situation that shifts the growth cycle to a longer-than- normal rest period. Because the range of causes is diverse—from injury or severe stress to response to drugs, severe chronic illness or infection, hypothyroidism, iron deficiency, or after physical stress such as surgery—telogen effluvium cannot be predicted to occur in one gender or another, one age group or another, except according to demographics for the underlying condition. Women between ages 40 and 70, however, are more affected by telogen effluvium than men, and typically shed a greater number of hairs in daily losses, sometimes by the handful. Because more women than men have thyroid disease, losses due to hypothyroidism, or as a result of a reaction to beta blockers used to treat hyperthyroidism or thyrotoxicosis, affect women more than men.

Cicatricial alopecia caused by damage to hair follicles and the scalp itself is a scarring form of alopecia with a range of causes such as infection, immunodeficiency, autoimmune disease, scalp trauma, and radiation therapy. Cicatricial alopecia can affect healthy individuals—men and women of all ages and all races. Approximately 3 percent of all cases of hair loss will be diagnosed as cicatricial alopecia. A type of primary cicatricial alopecia called *keratosis follicularis spinulosa decalvans* affects teenagers. A form called *central centrifugal alopecia* affects African-American individuals more than other races. *Frontal fibrosing alopecia* occurs in postmenopausal women. A form of primary cicatricial alopecia, an autoimmune disease called *chronic cutaneous lupus erythematosus*, develops in individuals with a family history of autoimmune diseases, indicating a genetic cause. As with telogen effluvium, in secondary cicatricial alopecia that stems from the presence of another illness, we can only predict who will be affected by the demographics for the underlying cause. Since the advent of the AIDS epidemic in the latter part of the twentieth century, more men currently have immunodeficiency than do women, and are more apt to develop alopecia from this known cause. However, women are affected more by autoimmune disease such as rheumatoid arthritis, lupus, and multiple sclerosis, and are therefore more subject to alopecia stemming from this cause. Obviously, we cannot accurately predict who will be affected by radiation therapy or scalp trauma such as burns or injuries.

Trichotillomania, a form of hair loss that is actually a behavior problem, occurs more often in females (90 percent) than in males, usually between ages 12 and 29, and occurs even more frequently in children younger than age 2, but the cases are milder and occur equally among boys and girls. Although many cases go unreported because of negative social aspects, it is estimated that 2.5 million people in the United States have trichotillomania, representing a prevalence rate of 1 percent in the whole population.

COMMON MISPERCEPTIONS ABOUT WOMEN AND HAIR LOSS

We've just seen how many women are affected by hair loss. I had no idea when my own hair loss developed that 20 percent of all women had some degree of thinning hair during their lifetime—it has been kept a secret, by the women themselves and within society. And the medical community has even helped to a certain extent. This is largely the result of the fact that men's hair loss or pattern baldness is noticeable in our society and, because women's hair loss is generally diffuse rather than patterned, it is less noticeable. In addition, women can often disguise the losses with hairstyling. The conclusion has been that women's hair loss is extremely rare. If we don't see it, it's not there.

The assumption that very few women are affected by hair loss, combined with the impression that balding is so common in men that it has become socially acceptable, has led to the social unacceptability of women's hair loss. This notion has made it especially difficult for women to face hair loss when it occurs, producing such an emotional impact that revealing the hair loss is taboo, even when treatment could possibly reverse the condition. When it was widely publicized that the hair growth medication Propecia was approved for men but not for women, this, too, gave a signal that women's hair loss was not a target for drug development, and therefore must not be much of a problem. Or, an even worse conclusion, that medical researchers and the medical community didn't take women's hair loss seriously. (Note: Propecia is a registered trademark of Merck & Company.)

Happily, these perceptions are gradually diminishing as hair loss in women becomes a topic that we can talk about and for which we can seek help. The April 2008 issue of *Vogue* magazine had a wonderfully honest article about a beautiful, talented woman who discovered she was losing hair and how she and other women she knew were able to deal with hair loss. The emotional aspects were discussed along with a range of treatments, and readers learned how several women proceeded through diagnosis and treatment to satisfying results. Not-so-satisfying results were discussed, too.

Also in 2008, one of a group of outstanding physicians recognized by *New York Magazine* was Dr. Robert M. Bernstein of the Center for Hair Restoration in New York City (see Resources), a physician hair replacement specialist and surgeon who performs surgical hair restoration, including hair transplantation, with demonstrated good results. Centers like Dr. Bernstein's are cropping up all over the country, treating men and women regularly. New drug therapies are also in development, and it is predicted that someday cloning techniques will be used to produce new follicles for transplantation (see "Making Headway in Cloning Hair," chapter 6). As attitudes and therapies change, the topic is fast becoming "hair loss," not male or female hair loss necessarily, even with certain recognized clinical differences.

WHO TREATS ALOPECIA?

Although primary care physicians may often be the first to confront their patients' hair loss issues, they will recognize alopecia as a complex multifactorial condition and may be reluctant to treat either its medical or psychological aspects, referring patients instead to a dermatologist or physician hair restoration specialist. Some patients do not seek help for suspected hair loss or balding, feeling hesitant about raising hair loss as a health issue, especially when they may feel it is primarily a cosmetic issue affecting only their personal appearance. When the topic of hair loss *is* broached by patients, family practitioners often share their patients' general embarrassment about the issue, even knowing that it's truly a health issue and a treatable condition. When asked, some physicians readily describe their own lack of awareness about just how many women suffer hair loss, or how devastating the experience can be for some patients. Because hair loss is a skin condition and not a hair condition per se, and because frequent and significant psychological and psychosocial aspects are known to accompany hair loss, primary care physicians may refer male and female patients with signs of alopecia to dermatologists for medical care, and to psychologists or psychotherapists for associated psychosocial aspects, rather than to begin treating the symptoms themselves. Still other individuals will go first to a hair clinic or salon to seek cosmetic solutions rather than seeking medical help.

So, who should you see about hair loss then? Years ago, no single type of medical specialist dealt exclusively with hair loss conditions—we didn't have many hair loss specialists. Dermatologists are the leading experts simply because follicles are part of skin surfaces and are often the source of the hair loss problem. If you are not yet certain that you have a specific type of hair loss condition, you can start with your family doctor or general practitioner unless you are already seeing a specialist about a chronic or acute condition such as diabetes, autoimmune disease (e.g., lupus, rheumatoid arthritis, or polymyalgia), or a thyroid condition such as Hashimoto's disease (also an autoimmune disease) or hypothyroidism. If you are taking a medication known to affect hair growth, it makes sense to first consult the doctor who prescribed the medication. Otherwise, you can go directly to a dermatologist who already has the knowledge to diagnose scalp and hair conditions. Or you can set up a consultation with a hair restoration clinic with a staff of physician hair restoration specialists who will be able to advise you about both medical and cosmetic approaches to your problem. You can get help finding such a specialist by contacting the International Society of Hair Restoration Surgery and the American Hair Loss Society (AHLS), among other organizations (see Resources).

While you are reading this book, you may likely discover a type of alopecia that seems to resemble your own condition. Rather than trying to diagnose yourself, however, it's essential that you consult your physician or a dermatologist or physician hair restoration specialist as soon as you think you're shedding or losing hair, or if your hair seems to be thinning, or when hair loss becomes distinctly noticeable in one or more areas of your scalp. If you experience burning or itching of the scalp, even without noticeable hair loss, it's still a reason to have your physician, a dermatologist, or a hair specialist examine the scalp for a condition that could possibly lead to hair loss.

Early diagnosis and early treatment, as with other clinical conditions, may increase your chances of stopping the hair loss.

CHOOSING A DOCTOR TO DIAGNOSE AND TREAT HAIR LOSS

Your choice of a medical professional is as personal as your hair loss problem. Even though you may have some idea of what you'd like to accomplish with treatment, and what you want your hair to look like *after* treatment, you'll need lots of guidance along the way to a happy result. That's why finding the physician who will diagnose your condition and advise you about your treatment options is the most critical step once you've decided to seek help. Although information alone can't promise you a good result, you are entitled to interview prospective doctors and see who gives you the answers that make you most comfortable. Here are some things you might want to consider asking in your search for a doctor:

- From what medical school and in what year did the physician graduate and what type of degree does he or she have (MD, DO, or ND, for example)?
- How many years has the physician been in practice?
- What is the physician's specialty (such as medical, surgical, dermatology, plastic surgery, or other)? How many years in that specialty? Is he or she board certified in the specialty?
- Is hair restoration the physician's primary practice currently? How long has the physician been specializing in hair restoration?
- How many hair transplant procedures has he or she performed? How many per month?
- Are the physician's patients satisfied with the results of treatment— especially the type of treatment you are considering? Would you be able to talk to someone who has had a particular procedure?
- Does the physician seem willing to discuss your treatment options openly?
- Does the physician pay attention and show interest in what you want from your treatment?

- Are costs for the procedures and treatments outlined for you in print and are payment options explained?
- And finally, are you comfortable with this physician and were your questions answered to your satisfaction?

Don't be afraid to ask questions. You may be in this patient/physician relationship for a significant amount of time and you want it to be a good one with good results. Meanwhile, you can use the information presented in *Women and Alopecia: Managing Unexplained Hair Loss* to give you some helpful background, and help you to be better prepared to discuss your problem with the doctor you finally select.

CHAPTER 2

WHAT IS HAIR AND HOW DOES IT GROW?

Hair chemistry, normal healthy hair follicles, phases of growth and rest, genetic/hereditary components, genetic defects that affect hair growth, relationship between hormones and hair growth (hair loss after menopause and childbirth, oral contraceptives and hair loss), common conditions that can lead to hair loss

WHAT IS HAIR, ANYWAY—AND WHY DOESN'T IT HURT WHEN WE CUT IT?

Hair loss can be frustrating and upsetting, not only for those women who experience it but for the physicians who are asked to explain it. Even though hair loss is a universal problem that has been around as long as humans have, the diagnosis and treatment of hair loss conditions has not always been a priority, leaving both physicians and patients wanting more information and more options. Understanding the functional aspects (physiology) of normal hair growth could help you identify your own hair loss problem, and understanding what can go wrong with the hair growth cycle may point to conditions that have caused or contributed to your problem. Once you have some hair chemistry knowledge and a general idea of how hair grows—or doesn't—you will be that much closer to getting the medical care you need and identifying your options.

Although you may not need to fully understand the chemical makeup of your hair to understand hair loss, having some background could definitely help you prepare for that first talk with your doctor and subsequent diagnosis and treatment of your problem. The normal hair growth cycle is a complex system that's quite amazing, considering the size of an individual hair. But if you have the patience to read through a basic review of hair chemistry, you may learn how and why the hair responds to various substances in the body— some that occur naturally, and some that are added from the environment.

You may already know that your hair is basically protein in nature. Hair is actually about 88 percent protein, made up of hard, fibrous proteins called *keratins*. Fingernails, by the way, are also composed of keratin. Keratins occur in polypeptide chains (*poly* = "many" and *peptide* = "broken down protein") of individual amino acids, which are the principle proteins in the body. Since we don't make the components of proteins on our own, we have to get the raw materials from the proteins we eat—beans, legumes, meat, fish, eggs, and dairy products, among others. We digest consumed proteins, break them down into individual amino acids, and then rebuild amino acid proteins as we need them. Getting back to hair, many amino acids join together to form polypeptide chains—many broken-down proteins—with peptide bonds between each of the individual amino acids. The chains are of different lengths and include a different order of amino acids to form each protein, including keratin, insulin, and collagen—proteins you have undoubtedly heard of, whether you knew they were proteins or not. In scientific terms, the keratin protein found in our hair is called the *alpha helix* and it looks like a coil (helix), with three and a half amino acids at each turn of the coil. Three alpha helices then wind around each other in a fibril structure called a *protofibril*. Nine of these gather around at least two more protofibrils to form a stronger cablelike fibril called a *microfibril*. Covering this cable, which now contains hundreds of microfibrils, is a protein-type coating containing sulfur. The entire bundle is called a *macrofibril*, which finally gives us the *cortex* (main body) of a single hair fiber. It's hard to believe there is that much happening in a hair fiber, but just as in electronic equipment, the more that is going on, the greater the number of things that can break down.

There's even more activity going on within a single hair than maintaining protein composition. In its normal state, for example, which is being flexible but not so flexible that it could be called "stretched," the hair structure is maintained by the bonding of alpha helices (plural of *helix*) in the cortex layer. Some of the interesting bonds between each and every alpha helix give hair its characteristics, including:

Hydrogen bond—responsible for elasticity or "stretchability" of the hair. Hydrogen bonds let us wash our hair with water, temporarily stretching each hair and then allowing it to go back to its original shape—thank goodness. Besides giving hair 50 percent or more of its elasticity, the hydrogen bond also gives hair 35 percent of its strength.

Salt bond—responsible for another 35 percent of hair's strength and even more elasticity. A salt bond is formed by the transfer of electrons from one chain of an amino group to the side chain of an acidic amino acid. The salt bond is called an ionic bond, representing an attraction between a positive and negative charge.

Cystine bond, also called the sulfur bond or disulfide bond—responsible for hair's toughness or resistance to abrasion. It's what allows us to perm our hair, among other things. The bond is formed by linkages between amino acid residues and is located across (or perpendicular to) the axis of the hair and between the polypeptide chains, actually holding the twisted hair fibers in place.

Sugar bond—responsible for giving hair toughness and endurance, this bond is between an amino acid side chain and an acidic amino group, somewhat like the salt bond. However, it is perpendicular to the hair's axis and in its function contributes moisture to the hair. Unlike the salt bond, it contributes little strength.

Surrounding this complex structure is the cuticle of the hair, which is composed of dead cells. Yes, the outer hair that we actually see on our head is made up of dead cells, somewhat like the bark of a tree, which is also a dead outer coating on a living thing. (Some people believe that because the outer cuticle is dead, we cannot feel anything when hair is cut. The only feeling, and it's slight, may occur at the follicle.) Dead cells or not, the cuticle is like an outer protective sleeve for the hair fiber, and microscopically, the dead cells are seen to overlap like fish scales, which helps explain the cuticle's overall strength. Without the cuticle, the hair fiber is much more vulnerable to possible external damage from chemicals or overprocessing—all the things we do to our hair to "improve" its appearance. Ironically, if we expect perms and straighteners, bleaches and coloring agents to work as we wish, the cuticle must first be opened up to allow the chemicals to get to the cortex of the hair and alter the chemical bonds in the hair structure or alter pigment. It's fairly easy to see why, without protection of the cuticle, excessive exposure to chemicals or the presence of highly concentrated chemicals could damage the cortex or weaken the hair fiber itself, neither of which is as strong as the cuticle. After prolonged, repeated, or improper processing of any kind, damaged hair can break off at the follicle and the result is … alopecia.

Finally, a canal in the center of the hair, in the midst of all the fibril layers, picks up and holds foreign debris that the body doesn't recognize as body cells or as usable material, including such things as heavy metals, synthetic chemicals, and medications, which will ultimately be excreted through the canal. You can see perhaps, the miracle of this hair chemistry, and how fortunate we are that foreign substances that could possibly destroy our hair are at least intended to be discharged. Understanding this, it's pretty clear that taking care of our hair requires more than shampoo and conditioner. We need to pay attention to what we put into our body.

Understanding hair chemistry may not be essential, but it does give us greater insight into some of the effects of our hair care and our exposure to foreign substances. We can understand better, for example, that the heat of blow dryers, curling irons, and heated rollers can potentially take away the already limited amount of moisture from our hair (remember the sugar bond?). We can more readily imagine the potential damage of chemicals in permanent wave processes, coloring agents, and hair relaxants, when we remember how hair gets its strength through microscopic and electronic bonds. Do you remember the cystine bond that allows us to curl our hair? And how strong the cuticle layer of our hair is, those dead cells on the outside of each hair? How will the cuticle stand up to potential mechanical damage from heavy brushing, brushing wet hair, pulling out knots, braiding, plaiting, dreads, cornrows, or even repeated combing? And think about the cleansing function of the canal at the center of each tiny hair. Will it pick up and excrete all the chemicals we put into our body—the drug therapies, over-the-counter medications, mercury, lead, and pesticides from the environment? We can only hope it will work as planned. Or, we could take responsibility for reducing unnecessary chemical exposure and help protect our hair and our bodies.

HOW DOES YOUR HAIR GROW?

Hair grows about six inches each year in healthy adults, which means about half an inch of growth each month. This varies among individuals, of course, and the figures we give here are averages. About 100,000 hairs can be found on the average adult scalp at any given time, regardless of gender or race. Hair also has a turnover rate, a regular cycle of hair growth and loss. In most individuals, about 100 to 150 hairs, give or take, are shed naturally each day, while even more can be shed during shampooing. This shedding is absolutely normal and losses are not usually noticeable on your head because replacement growth is a continuous process in normal, healthy individuals. There is no need to worry about the hairs you may find on your sink, tub, and pillow—they're usually nothing to be concerned about unless you see handfuls at a time.

Hairs are about 0.02 to 0.04 mm thick. It takes about 20 to 50 hairs to equal a millimeter. Healthy hair can actually be as strong as steel wire and, if so, it is said to take a force of 60 kg or more to break a single hair. Healthy scalp hairs will live two to six years on the head before they are shed and replaced. Depending on an individual's rate of hair growth, which in turn depends on age, diet, overall health, and hair care, waist-length hair would take about six years of growth since the hairs' lifetime is what controls the maximum possible hair length. In other words, if the lifecycle of your hair is only two years, you will not likely be able to grow waist-length hair.

The duration of hair growth cycles varies with different body areas. Eyebrows, eyelashes, facial hair, body hair, and pubic hair are generally shorter hairs with longer growth cycles. That is, it takes longer to grow and replace them, and therefore they remain short. Imagine if they grew as quickly as scalp hair, the earth would look like the *Planet of the Apes*. Men with a mustache and/or beard may notice that these hairs grow more rapidly in the summer than in the winter, a rather odd situation since hair helps prevent loss of body heat. Research has shown that the hair on our head and in beards has peak growth in autumn months, slows down in the coldest months, and picks up again come spring and summer. This is a bit odd, too, since many people prefer shorter hair in hotter months, thinking it will keep the head and neck cooler.

How many of the 100,000 hairs on your head do you have to lose before you notice it? And when will it become noticeable to someone else? When you first begin to notice thinning of the hair on your head, it can simply mean that more hair has fallen out that can be replaced in a normal period of time. This can indicate a hair growth problem, true, but it may not be alopecia. It's when lost hair is not replaced at all that the result is balding. Thinning of hair can also indicate that the hairs themselves have become thinner, having a smaller cylindrical shape or diameter, which allows more of your scalp to be seen. Other changes may include softer texture of the hairs, shorter hair length associated with a longer growth period for each new hair, and color changes—sometimes with hairs actually becoming almost colorless.

But that's about thinning hair rather than *losing* hair. To answer the question about how many hairs you have to lose before you notice it, the consensus among hair experts and dermatologists is that half your hair will need to be lost, and at that point, you may be the first to see it but will surely not be the *only* one who sees it.

HAIR UP CLOSE

The body of a single hair is called a *hair shaft*. Under a microscope you would see that each hair has an outer layer of cells—dead cells, if you remember hair chemistry—that are closely woven to protect the delicate shaft. This outer covering as we learned in hair chemistry is called the *cuticle*, just like the halfmoon at the base of your fingernails. It's what gives our hair its shine by reflecting light. If it is damaged in any way, such as by too many treatments like permanents or coloring, the cell layers raise up and expose the under layers of the cortex, which releases needed moisture and dries out the hair. The raised cells of multiple hairs will then grab onto each other, producing the "frizz" and tangles we don't want. Shampoos, conditioners, and conditioning treatments are then needed to calm and smooth the hair shaft again, so that hair shines and behaves well.

AT THE ROOT OF HAIR GROWTH—THE FOLLICLE

How does hair growth begin? Hair follicles begin to form in the fetus during a woman's first three months of pregnancy (first trimester) and are almost fully formed at birth. The follicles you were born with are the ones you'll have throughout your lifetime. Follicles are never replaced, even if they become damaged, and no new follicles ever develop. In the fetus, however, follicles will develop all over the body—scalp, face, arms, underarms, legs, back, chest, belly, pubic region—wherever hair is likely to grow. We can guess that there are more follicles on the scalp than anywhere else, consequently resulting in greater hair growth in most individuals. The follicles themselves will change as we age, including their size, color, shape, and types of activity related to hair growth. The average number of hairs on a normal scalp range from about 90,000 to 150,000, depending on the number of follicles. And, believe it or not, the number of follicles we have corresponds to our hair color. Blonds, for example, may have 140,000 hairs; people with brown hair will have about 105,000; and redheads have the least, about 90,000. And why does color influence number? Each hair color is associated with a different size follicle and different size hairs, with the hair size related to the diameter or caliber of the hair. Blond hair is finest and therefore more individual hairs cover the scalp; brown hair is midsize and thicker; and red hairs are thickest of all, with fewer hairs needed to cover the head.

A follicle observed under a microscope appears to be a tiny tube in the skin layers of the scalp, with an opening (*pore*) at the skin surface. Each follicle extends into the layers of skin, supported on each side by a muscle. These muscles are small ones, but just like larger muscles in the body, they can contract, causing hair to stand on end and the outer end of the follicle to protrude in a little mound we commonly call a goose bump. Each hair—or *hair shaft* as the body of the hair is called—grows from a root within a hair follicle, receiving nourishment from a network of tiny blood vessels. Also in the hair follicle is an oil-producing gland (*sebaceous gland*) that manufactures a substance (*sebum*) to remove dead skin cells from the scalp. Sebum also performs a conditioning function for the scalp and helps prevent loss of natural moisturizing fluid from the outer layer of skin. Hair follicles provide an optimum nourishing environment for the hair growth cycle. To maintain this environment for an individual's lifetime, the body must also maintain the follicles' complex structure, replacing their cell walls rapidly and continuously. It takes a healthy follicle to continue producing healthy hair. You will see how important this is as we learn more about the hair growth cycle.

Diagram 1: Hair Follicle in Growth Phase

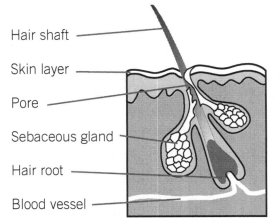

The normal hair growth cycle of the scalp and other body parts is made up of three phases of follicle activity: the anagen phase, catagen phase, and telogen phase. These phases vary in duration in each area of the body, but even though follicle activity cycles for different periods of time, the same growth characteristics are maintained in each area of hair growth. You will also begin to notice as you work your way through the book that the three phases of follicle activity are reflected in the names of the different types of alopecia, providing clues as to which phase has been affected. The discussion below is devoted primarily to growth cycles of hair follicles on the scalp, not the rest of the body.

Anagen phase—period of active hair growth; about 85 to 90 percent of scalp follicles are growing in anagen at any given time for all healthy individuals. Follicles stay in an anagen phase of consistent growth for up to three years, although this can range from two to six years among different individuals. In this phase of growth, the matrix cells of each hair follicle are engaged in vigorous reproductive activity (mitosis)—that is, dividing and reproducing themselves. Each hair will have a long, indented root with an outer root sheath covering it. Hairs will be pigmented. Toward the end of the anagen phase, pigmentation will decrease close to the follicle.

Catagen phase—after anagen, 2 to 3 percent of follicles pass into a transitional period of regression, in which there is little or no growth activity, but hair remains healthy with no hair loss or lack of growth that we can notice. Hair in the catagen phase is not engaged in mitosis or cell division and reproduction. Follicles in their sheath of connective tissue move up toward the outer layer of skin (epidermis), preparing for the telogen or resting phase.

Telogen phase—up to 15 percent of follicles will undergo a period of dormancy, or rest, for about three months, during which no growth of these hairs occurs. Again, because only a small percentage of hairs are involved, we don't notice any loss or lack of growth in a normal rest phase of the cycle. Telogen hairs rest until follicles decide spontaneously to return to anagen, forced out by growing hairs coming up underneath.

At the end of the telogen phase, dead hair is released from the skin and a firm white nodule or *bulb* can be found at each follicle, the end point of the external hair that has been ejected. The cycle then begins again for that follicle. The return to the anagen phase will not happen consistently across the scalp, and the length of each phase and the length of the whole cycle will vary according to the location on the scalp and the individual's age. Although follicles will cycle for different periods on each body area, on the scalp, the anagen phase of growth activity averages about 1,000 days (total period can range from two to five years), with only two to four weeks for the transient catagen phase, and an average of about 100 days (range of three to four months) for the resting or telogen phase. The majority of hair follicles at any particular time will be in anagen. There's also a difference in the percentages of anagen and telogen hairs in scalp hair growth between men and women: at any given time, females have a ratio of about 85 percent anagen to 15 percent telogen hairs, while males have a ratio of about 81–90 percent anagen to 10–19 percent telogen hairs (depending on the individual, the ratio will vary, but obviously will add up to 100 percent!)

CLASSIFYING HAIR LOSS ACCORDING TO STAGES OF GROWTH AND REST

There are many types of hair loss—we saw the most common ones in chapter 1 and a more thorough explanation is coming up in chapter 3. However, there are ways to group them other than under either *hair loss with healthy follicles or hair loss with damaged follicles*. We can use the anagen and telogen stages of growth and rest in which hairs are shed but follicles are unharmed, outlined briefly as follows:

Anagen Phase Hair Problem

Anagen effluvium—impaired reproductive or growth activity following toxic exposure (e.g., chemotherapy, radiation, or poisons) or severe inflammation of matrix in anagen phase.

Telogen Phase Hair Problem

Telogen effluvium—early, excessive shedding from normal resting follicles regardless of the trigger or causative underlying illness.

This classification describes only two forms of hair loss; however, and we must rely on the characteristics of all forms in order to understand their causes, treatments, and possible outcomes.

41

GENETICALLY INFLUENCED HAIR SHAFT DEFECTS THAT RESULT IN HAIR LOSS

Genetic defects can sometimes cause abnormal formation of hair fibers by hair follicles. One of the results of this genetic defect can be *loose hair syndrome* (loose anagen syndrome), a condition in which the hairs of the head are easily pulled out from the hair follicle. It is sometimes found in young children, girls more than boys, whose hair doesn't seem to grow and remains baby-fine and thin over the entire scalp. The back of the head that touches the pillow at night may lose hair more rapidly and begin to bald. Although this condition often corrects by itself as the child passes age five or so, if it persists into adulthood, hair loss may be more noticeable. The cause is believed to be the root sheath that normally protects the hair shaft does not adhere to the shaft and is not properly anchored within the follicle. No effective treatments are known for loose hair syndrome and the precise genetic pathway has not been described. Because it so rarely occurs in adults, and is not technically alopecia, it is not discussed further in this book.

Another genetically based hair condition is *monilethrix*, a condition in which nodes and constrictions along the hair fiber make a single hair resemble a string of beads. The beading results in weakening the hair fiber, making it brittle and causing breakage, sometimes resulting in diffuse hair loss. The condition is most often diagnosed in children and teenagers and is found to run in families. It can improve on its own or can continue throughout adult life. It is not a form of alopecia even though it may result in hair loss. For this reason, it is not discussed further in this book.

HORMONES AND HAIR GROWTH—HAIR LOSS AFTER MENOPAUSE AND CHILDBIRTH

How and why male pattern baldness affects women in the first place may seem implausible, but women experience the same type of hair loss that is common in men—not as extensively or as noticeably, of course, and usually occurring at the time of menopause or in the years after. What is the relationship? The name *androgenetic*, as in *androgenetic alopecia* or *androgenic alopecia*, tells the story. A genetic relationship is part of the cause, and the other part is the presence of androgens (male hormone such as testosterone), which have been shown by researchers to influence the shutting down of hair production in men or women whose genetic profile—the genes inherited from both parents—predisposes them to this type of loss. No specific genes have been implicated as an actual cause, but researchers believe that several genes may contribute to pattern baldness, calling the condition *polygenetic*.

Androgen receptors are found in the hair follicles of men and women—androgen-sensitive follicles are found on the top of the head and androgen-independent follicles are found on the sides and back of the head. These locations actually give us some clues about the characteristics of pattern baldness as it occurs in men and women. When androgens are present, genes that control the active growing stage or anagen phase of hair growth shorten this part of the growth/loss cycle, resulting in subsequent shrinking (miniaturization) of hair follicles, which eventually changes larger, pigmented hairs (terminal hairs) into shorter, finer (*vellus* or velluslike hairs) and less overall growth. Although androgens are male hormones, women do have them in lower levels. In women, they are surpassed by estrogen levels during most of women's adult years, and estrogens don't miniaturize hair follicles. However, during and after menopause, women lose estrogen in the presence of increased androgens, which tips their hormone balance. Next step—hair loss. Hair growth is particularly sensitive to fluctuations in hormones, but some women seem to be protected, either for genetic reasons or because women have an enzyme (aldactose) that converts androgens to estrogens, which don't miniaturize hair follicles. Nevertheless, a large percentage of menopausal women (up to 87 percent according to results of studies) will notice some hair thinning as they grow older and may resort to using volumizing shampoos and conditioners or develop a certain hairstyle to compensate. Although it occurs primarily after menopause, in some women loss of hair can begin as early as young adulthood or puberty, either noticeably or not. When premenopausal women were studied, up to 87 percent were found to have some degree of hair thinning considered to be androgenetic alopecia.

During pregnancy, the percentage of hair follicles that are in the telogen rest phase decreases progressively, especially in the last three months of pregnancy. As hormones change after childbirth, women may lose hair for two or three months, primarily because the interrupted hormone cycle during pregnancy has also interrupted the hair growth cycle, preventing normal hair loss and replacement. This is usually considered to be a form of telogen effluvium resulting from the sudden change in hormones after childbirth; almost as quickly as it appeared, it readily corrects itself when hormone balance returns. (See "Androgenetic Alopecia" and "Telogen Effluvium," chapter 3.)

As a point of interest in this discussion of hair replacement growth, after loss of hair has occurred and hair growth begins to resume, non-pigmented hair may replace pigmented hair, which is the process that causes gray hairs. We know that some people turn gray before others—it's all a matter of when androgenetic hair loss begins and whether pigmented hair is replaced by non-pigmented or gray hairs.

ORAL CONTRACEPTIVES AND ANDROGENS

Since the oral contraceptive—or "the pill," as it has been called—was introduced in the 1960s, it has become the most accepted form of birth control among millions of women. Since that time, we have also learned that oral contraceptives are a common source of hair loss, functioning as described in this chapter's discussion of hormones and hair growth. This is because of the intentional changes in estrogen and progestin levels, or sometimes in progestin alone, as a result of the pill's mechanism for suppressing ovulation. Some women can be especially sensitive to the hormone changes or are genetically susceptible to the androgenetic form of hair loss (androgenetic alopecia) and these women are more likely to experience some degree of hair loss while taking the pill or for several weeks after they stop taking the pill.

The American Hair Loss Association (AHLA) (see Resources) advises women who are taking the pill to evaluate their genetic susceptibility before they start. (Ask yourself: Does hair loss run in my family?) If they are likely to be more susceptible because hair loss runs in the family, they are advised by the AHLA to use only a low-androgen birth control pill or a nonhormonal form of birth control. Progestin implants, skin patches, vaginal rings, and hormone injections are associated with a higher risk of causing hair loss in women who are sensitive to hormones or who have a history of hair loss in their families. Manufacturers of oral contraceptives must make the androgen content of their products known to users; it can usually be found in the package insert. Your doctor may also have this information or can readily get it before you fill your prescription for oral contraceptives.

COMMON CONDITIONS AT THE ROOT OF HAIR LOSS

We now know that heredity, or genetics, hormones, and aging can cause hair loss. What else could be responsible? Actually, a wide range of explanations for hair loss have been proposed, researched, and confirmed, including conditions that are traumatic to the body or that deplete it's nutritional reserves, and diseases that upset body metabolism—the way we assimilate nutrients from our diets, and process and distribute them to maintain normal, healthy energy levels and body processes. Common conditions at the root of hair loss, besides heredity/genetics, hormones, and aging, include:

- Iron deficiency
- Thyroid disease (hypothyroidism)
- Poor blood circulation
- Acute illnesses that disturb body processes and deplete nutritional stores
- Surgery—a form of trauma that disturbs the body
- Exposure to radiation—whether diagnostic, accidental, or environmental
- Scalp or skin infections—bacterial or fungal
- Skin disease that may damage hair follicles
- Sudden weight loss that depletes the body's reserves
- High fever
- Diabetes
- Autoimmune disease—when the immune system attacks hair follicles as if they were foreign (See "Alopecia Areata," chapter 3)
- Certain medications (see chapter 4 for more details)
- Chemotherapeutic drugs that destroy cells (cytotoxic or cytostatic drugs) or suppress the immune system (immunosuppressants)
- Stress and stressful events
- Poor diet, poor nutritional status
- Vitamin and mineral deficiencies (zinc, biotin)
- Vitamin A excess from overconsumption (more than 100,000 IU daily, long term)

Any of these conditions can increase the risk for hair loss in women. It is the physician's task to study your entire health history, your family history of illness and hair loss, and all of your symptoms, and then to perform diagnostic testing and determine why you are losing your hair. It can be a long, arduous process to make a diagnostic decision between one type of hair loss and another. The types of hair loss that may be triggered by the conditions listed on page 45 are discussed more fully in chapter 3. How these hair loss conditions are diagnosed is discussed in chapter 4.

TYPES OF ALOPECIA: SIGNS, SYMPTOMS, AND CAUSES

Types of hair loss, range of symptoms, types of treatment recommended, likely outcomes, possible complications, the importance of early diagnosis

SIGNS, SYMPTOMS, AND CAUSES OF HAIR LOSS

Hair loss is not as simple as just losing hair, shedding hair, or thinning of hair. As you are beginning to learn, hair loss is associated with a broad range of conditions—some sources say over two hundred possible causes—some directly responsible for hair loss and some existing as an underlying condition. Add stress to this mix, and a perfect climate has been created in which alopecia can develop.

Androgenetic alopecia (AGA) is statistically the most common form of alopecia, whether manifesting in men as male pattern baldness or in women as female androgenetic alopecia (female AGA), or female pattern baldness. Although society, and men themselves to a certain extent, has more or less accepted the genetically influenced baldness that we commonly see in men, female AGA that leads to significant thinning or actual baldness seems to carry a far greater stigma and far greater psychosocial effect, begging the attention of clinicians and researchers to develop solutions. Meanwhile, another whole range of nonandrogenetic alopecias are being diagnosed and treated, each with the same possible devastating effect of losing hair.

Telogen effluvium (TE), either acute or chronic, is the most prevalent nonandrogenetic alopecia seen by dermatologists and the second most common form of alopecia. *Chronic telogen effluvium* (CTE) occurs primarily in middle-aged women. The acute forms of TE are caused by so many different underlying conditions that they fit most closely under the phrase "unexplained alopecia." An experienced diagnostician, whether your own doctor or a dermatologist, will be able to identify the underlying condition, which will be the first step in identifying appropriate treatment. Two recognized types of telogen effluvium encountered in women, for example, are caused by iron deficiency and thyroid disease (hypothyroidism). Effective treatment of the underlying condition will usually reverse hair shedding. Not all forms of telogen effluvium, however, are as easily identified and treated.

The third most common alopecia, another nonandrogenetic form, is autoimmune alopecia, or alopecia areata (AA), which affects 2 percent of the population, occurring more often in women than in men. This form of alopecia is classified as an autoimmune disorder, but development of the disorder is known to be triggered by acute or chronic stress.

Chemically induced and physically induced causes also damage the hair. Among these causes are overprocessing, cuticle stripping, aggressive brushing and back combing, and physical abuse of the hair fiber that may flake away the protective cuticle. Hair can break off at the follicle with any one of these harsh treatments and the result is alopecia.

The list of types of hair loss goes on, each form of alopecia stemming from different causes, producing different signs and symptoms that are addressed with different treatments, and resulting in a range of possible outcomes (prognoses). The main forms are discussed below, each with a set of causes, symptoms, treatments, and possible outcomes.

ANDROGENETIC ALOPECIA (AGA)

First a word about the various terms used to describe this most common form of alopecia, including alopecia genetica, androgenic alopecia, female pattern hair loss (PHL), and female androgenetic alopecia (female AGA). Because female AGA rarely results in the significant baldness characteristic of male pattern baldness, I prefer the term *female androgenetic alopecia* (female AGA) to *female pattern baldness*, and will primarily use this term and the term *androgenetic alopecia* in discussion. Be prepared to see any of the terms tossed about freely in other print or electronic discussions of female AGA; they're all referring to the genetic form of alopecia that affects nearly all women, especially postmenopausal women.

Androgenetic alopecia (AGA) is the most common form of hair loss in both men and women, stemming from progressive shortening of the anagen phase in hair growth cycles. If we take apart the name *androgenetic*, we learn that the condition derives partly from genetic sources such as genes inherited from either side of an individual's family. It's also related to the presence of a specific male hormone or androgen, (dihydrotestosterone), or to androgen excess (hyperandrogenism). Dihydrotestosterone (DHT) is a more potent form of testosterone that results when testosterone is converted by 5-alpha-reductase, an enzyme found in hair follicles. Follicles on the top of the scalp are typically androgen sensitive and on the sides and back of the head are androgen independent. The presence of testosterone and DHT decreases the size—or miniaturizes—follicles that are sensitive to androgens. The result is thinner and shorter hairs emerging from androgen-sensitive hair follicles. Male pattern baldness occurs in men with androgen excess or too much DHT in the scalp follicles; men who do not inherit the type of 5-alpha-reductase enzyme found in follicles do not produce DHT in follicles and do not develop androgenetic alopecia.

Female androgenetic alopecia is not a direct result of androgen excess as it is in men, although androgen excess does occur in some women, producing very different results than in men. In women, AGA or pattern hair loss results from the complex process in which androgens shorten the anagen phase of growth starting as early as puberty. As in men, when androgen-sensitive follicles become miniaturized, the result will be smaller, thinner hairs (referred to medically as vellus hairs or velluslike hairs) and general thinning, sometimes over the entire scalp. Not all women, however, have this sensitivity to androgens. The ones who do will notice that their hair is thinning and some may also notice female symptoms of androgen excess. Not to worry; there are ways to deal with all of these symptoms.

Classic pattern baldness corresponds to the distribution of follicles that are sensitive to the presence of androgen, which can vary from person to person. Female AGA pattern baldness is different from male pattern baldness. For one thing, it is considerably less obvious, and usually results in overall thinning of the front of the head above the forehead and hairline (frontal bone area) and the sides and top of the head (parietal bone area) while the hairline section of the front and the temple areas remain unchanged. In other words, women do not characteristically develop receding hairlines. By contrast, the hair loss pattern in men is described more or less as being in the shape of the letter M, with baldness at the temples—the classic receding hairline—and also with balding at the crown of the head, leaving hair on the sides and back. We have somewhat lost our sensitivity to these conditions in men. Because we see baldness so often in men, we give it little thought—it's just what happens as men age, and even before middle age in some men. Regardless of society's reaction, however, many men are extremely upset with their thinning hair or balding and eagerly seek solutions.

Androgen excess occurs most commonly in men, accounting for most of the various degrees of baldness we see among adult males. In women, androgen excess can produce various other conditions such as unwanted hair growth (hirsutism), ovarian abnormalities, irregular menstruation, infertility, and acne. Women who have none of these clinical symptoms will not usually have to undergo extensive hormone testing to identify AGA; it will be visually consistent with pattern hair loss in women. In other words, women who are seeing thinning of their hair, and are also seeing their skin become oily and breaking out, may have androgen excess. These women are converting estrogen to androgen and the androgens are affecting hair follicles, including oil production that leads to acne. It's all because they are genetically programmed to be sensitive to the presence of androgens and the conversion of estrogen is producing too many androgens. Often women with androgen excess (who do not know they are androgen sensitive) may be on a prescribed hormone regimen to reduce symptoms of menopause such as hot flashes. More estrogen takes care of the hot flashes well enough, but more estrogen is also available to convert to androgen, resulting in androgen excess. However, the problem is not *caused* by the estrogen replacement regimen in these cases; it's caused by underlying imbalances in the women's own hormone production.

Causes of Androgenetic Alopecia

Although androgenetic alopecia is the result of genetic and hormonal causes that negatively influence the hair growth cycle, it has also been shown that acute or chronic stress can be an aggravating factor in types of hair loss that stem from an endocrine, metabolic, or immunological nature as in female androgenetic alopecia. The combination of the underlying hormonal cause and stress can be a self-perpetuating problem, turning androgenetic hair loss into a chronic condition and complicating attempts to treat it. No actual gene or gene mutation has been identified in research studies to be the specific genetic cause of androgenetic alopecia and researchers think that because of the number of hair loss patterns, the age differences at onset, and different degrees of hair loss among women, that many genes may be at cause and other influences as well, including, of course, hormones and stress levels. On the hormone front, women are known to have lower levels of androgens than men and also known to have greater levels of an enzyme called *aromatase* that converts androgens to estrogens. These two factors may work together to help curb the tendency for women to develop AGA, since estrogens don't miniaturize hair follicles the way androgens do. Nevertheless, one study found that 87 percent of a large group of premenopausal women had some noticeable level of AGA (Venning and Dawber, 1988).

Symptoms of Androgenetic Alopecia

Women may have no other signs of androgenetic alopecia than "normal" generalized thinning of the hair during aging, which can allow the scalp to be visible through the thinner hair in more aggressive cases. Classic pattern baldness, in which thinning occurs in the center and frontal areas of the head but with little or no receding hair at the temples, may occur in women aged fifty and older, but will not always develop in women whose genetic makeup makes them susceptible. Women with severe androgenetic alopecia, however, may lose significant hair texture in the front of the head, with thinning being most noticeable in the frontal areas and on the sides of the head. The hair-line may remain unaffected. When severe, AGA can result in shorter hairs generally, and the resulting appearance can be a classic monk's hairstyle with a rim of hair around the periphery of the scalp and a relatively bald dome in the center, a rare pattern of loss in women and quite similar to male pattern baldness.

Dermatologists report that the typical clinical presentation of female AGA is diffuse thinning of the top and sides of the head with the frontal hairline remaining intact. A slight thinning or receding of the temple area may be seen in some women but a severe receding hairline is very unusual. If a deeper temple area recession of hair is seen along with thinning of the top and sides, acne, unwanted facial or body hair, and menstrual disorders of any kind, then severe androgen excess will likely be suspected.

Diagram 2: Progression of Female Pattern Alopecia

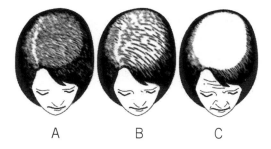

A   B   C

A. Hair part widening
B. Extensive widening of hair on top of head
C. Diffuse thinning over the crown of head with intact frontal hair

Treatment for Androgenetic Alopecia

Male pattern baldness and female pattern baldness are treated in much the same way except for sometimes restoring hormone balance in women who have androgen excess. Although pattern baldness manifests differently in men and women, the goal is the same, which is to restore hair growth. Many men accept their pattern hair loss even though they may seek hair replacement, and society has also more or less accepted it. Women generally find hair loss unacceptable and often seek treatment as soon as thinning or loss is noticed. Topical treatment with hair growth stimulants, such as minoxidil, is a common choice for women. And various surgical procedures such as the modern micro-graft transplants are gaining popularity as viable solutions for severe cases. Older surgeries such as scalp reduction and flaps are still available for women who are not candidates for transplantation. And low-level laser treatment has been shown to enhance hair growth, especially in cases of diffuse thinning that occurs with androgenetic alopecia in women. Nonprofessional hair clinics offer a variety of topical solutions, but results are notoriously poor in most cases, produce only short-lived results, or are prohibitively expensive. Some physicians, gynecologists especially, may help correct hair loss in women by regulating hormones when they are so out of balance that excess estrogen is being converted to androgens, and the androgen excess is causing hair loss. Chapter 5 will have more to say about the restoration of hormone balance as a treatment for female AHA.

Prognosis for Androgenetic Alopecia

Androgenetic alopecia in women is essentially a disorder of the normal hair growth cycle, and, according to expert opinion, may therefore be reversible in early stages if there are no complicating factors such as stress, underlying autoimmune or metabolic disease, or poor nutrition. Response to hair growth drugs can ultimately be successful if treatment is consistent, but individual response varies in relation to each woman's health status and genetic profile. In advanced or aggressive androgenetic alopecia, inflammation of the hair follicles may cause nonreversible damage to the follicular stem cell, resulting in a lack of response to standard treatment.

ADRENAL ANDROGENIC FEMALE PATTERN ALOPECIA

Similar to androgenetic alopecia, adrenal androgenic female pattern alopecia is characterized by chronic, diffuse hair loss in younger women (in their 20s and 30s), a condition that is usually progressive, affecting primarily the center of the scalp area. Studies of women who have the typical hair loss pattern of adrenal androgenic alopecia have been found to have elevated levels of a specific adrenal androgenic substance, called adrenal androgen dehydroepi-androsterone sulfate (DHEA-S), in their blood serum. Not much more is known about this hair loss condition except that a genetic cause is most likely. Treatment, if any, usually involves the same types of drug therapy or surgical treatment that have been effective for androgenetic alopecia.

ALOPECIA AREATA—AUTOIMMUNE ALOPECIA OR PATCHY HAIR LOSS

Alopecia areata is the third most common form of hair loss, developing as the result of an underlying autoimmune process. In autoimmune hair loss, a combination of antibodies, immune-system cells (T cells), and certain hormonelike proteins (cytokines) alter the normal follicular growth cycle, causing groups of follicles to enter the telogen, or rest, phase prematurely. As in other forms of autoimmune disease, the immune system has lost its ability to differentiate self-cells from non-self-cells and begins to treat a specific target within the body as though it were foreign. The specific target in alopecia areata is hair follicles all over the body. Varying amounts of hair can be lost in alopecia areata; hair can fall out in circular quarter-size areas here and there over the scalp, or it can involve larger areas and greater losses.

In rare instances, an individual may lose all hair on the scalp in alopecia areata (*alopecia areata totalis*) or even lose all body hair as well as scalp hair (*alopecia areata universalis*). One to 2 percent of the population has alopecia areata, affecting males and females equally. Although individuals of any age can be affected, the condition is most common in children and young adults; most individuals develop their first bald patch before they reach age twenty. As if losing hair were not enough, the condition may also be accompanied by other autoimmune diseases, as they tend to cluster, including autoimmune thyroid disease causing hypothyroidism or hyperthyroidism (Hashimoto's disease or Graves' disease), milky white patches on the skin (vitiligo, a skin condition also thought to be autoimmune in nature), and/or pernicious anemia.

Causes of Alopecia Areata

Acute or chronic stress can be a causative factor in types of hair loss that originally stem from an endocrine, metabolic, or immunological cause; this is believed to be the case in alopecia areata, because it is a form of autoimmune hair loss. A possible explanation is that an earlier illness that involves immune system response can sometimes cause the immune system to become hyperactive and produce too many killer T cells in preparation for fighting foreign cells; this activity can continue without actual provocation and result in autoimmune disease, but it is not known precisely how or why the immune system chooses to attack only hair follicles in alopecia areata, for example, or only joints in rheumatoid arthritis. Viruses have also been suggested as a possible trigger for autoimmune alopecia areata. Although alopecia areata may occur in individuals with thyroid disease, especially autoimmune Hashimoto's disease and Graves' disease, it is not believed to be caused by thyroid abnormalities per se. Researchers describe the coexistence of thyroid disease and alopecia areata as a factor of autoimmune conditions often occurring together because of the shared underlying immune system disorder.

Symptoms of Alopecia Areata

This form of alopecia typically begins with a single round or oval bare patch or a group of patches of well-defined bare areas; the condition can remain confined to a few bare patches or can eventually involve the entire scalp (alopecia totalis) or entire body (alopecia universalis) as discussed earlier.

Short, straight hairs of about several millimeters in length can be found standing around the outer edge of each patch, appearing microscopically as "exclamation points." Although inflammation is present at the roots of hair follicles, very little can be seen around the hair follicle openings on the scalp. Neither redness nor pain may be present. Some individuals, however, report tenderness, burning, and/or itchiness, and sometimes even pain, in the very beginning of the condition prior to noticing spots of hair loss. Nevertheless, patchy hair loss is usually the first sign.

Treatment for Alopecia Areata

Corticosteroid treatment is the most common approach for alopecia areata, using the application of corticosteroid cream on bald patches or injecting corticosteroid solutions into the balding areas. Steroid drugs may also be taken orally, but side effects restrict this approach to the most severe cases. Other types of chemicals are sometimes used directly on the scalp to provoke an allergic response that actually promotes hair growth. No generally effective treatment has yet shown consistently successful results in treating alopecia areata.

Wearing coverings such as wigs, hats, or scarves is recommended to protect the head from the elements—not a treatment exactly, but especially protective for alopecia areata, which is essentially a skin condition that has no cure. Hair loss can be in spots or the entire head but it doesn't grow back, so protection of the scalp is necessary.

Prognosis for Alopecia Areata

Alopecia areata usually reverses itself spontaneously six months to a year after it begins, although it's possible that new hair growth may be of a different color than the individual's normal hair color. Regrowth of bald patches can begin as early as one to three months after they first appear, but losses may be occurring at the same time on other areas of the scalp. Although remission is common (50 to 70 percent), many people experience recurrence (30 percent). The condition can become more extensive when it recurs, or symptoms can recur in cycles of loss and renewed growth. If the condition begins after puberty, begins to worsen noticeably, or continues much beyond one year, the prognosis is poorer. It is also poorer among children with Down syndrome or in families with a history of alopecia areata or autoimmune disease.

Individuals with total hair loss over the scalp (alopecia totalis) have a markedly reduced opportunity for long-term regrowth. Total loss of body hair (alopecia universalis) is extremely rare and when it does occur is usually noticed during childhood, not in adults.

TELOGEN EFFLUVIUM (TE)

Telogen effluvium can be acute or chronic, inflammatory or noninflammatory, and can begin abruptly or become noticed gradually. It is described as increased shedding of scalp hair, or diffuse scalp hair thinning, and more than other forms of alopecia falls into the catch-all category of "unexplained hair loss." More typically, however, if it occurs abruptly as an acute condition, it follows some obvious trauma or insult to the body such as a disease or response to surgery or reaction to a medication. An idiopathic form, meaning one that appears on its own with no apparent underlying cause, occurs primarily in middle-aged women and is called *chronic telogen effluvium* (CTE). This form can easily be confused with female androgenetic alopecia, although it doesn't show up as the typical AGA pattern hair loss involving scalp hair on the front (over frontal bone) and sides (over parietal bone) of the head. Acute telogen effluvium has a wide range of possible acquired causes, with stress shown to be an important influential or complicating factor even when it is not the direct cause.

TE occurs as an overall reduction in the number of scalp hairs. This reduction develops when normal phases of growth and rest are disrupted, and a disproportionate rest phase prevents a significant number of hairs from growing. The disrupted phase can also be the anagen or growth phase, resulting in hair loss described as *anagen effluvium*, the type of hair loss we see in chemotherapy or some other types of drug reactions (see "Anagen Effluvium," page 63). In TE, literally handfuls of hair are not being replaced during the imbalance between distribution of hair follicles in the growth phase (anagen) and an excess of follicles in the resting phase (telogen). The word *effluvium* means "outflow" and *telogen effluvium* essentially means "too much telogen." TE is also called *traumatic alopecia* because the shifts in growth and rest phases can follow a traumatic event, severe stress, acute illness with fever, or reaction to the use of certain medications. The traumatic event will typically have occurred several months prior to noticing excess shedding or a disruption in hair growth.

Three distinct triggers can lead to telogen effluvium:

1. A shock, environmental or physical, to the hair follicles in the growth phase so that they revert to a rest phase, resulting in excess shedding of hair. This form of TE can occur rapidly and hair shedding will be noticed as early as a month after the shock. The condition will last up to six months and normal hair growth will usually resume within a year. Triggers for this form of TE can be a traumatic experience or event such as an automobile accident or the death of a loved one, severe stress, or a physical shock such as high fever, surgery, sudden hormone changes after childbirth, or acute reaction to a medication.

2. Hair follicles in the normal rest phase continue in that phase without switching to the growth phase after a two-month period. This form of TE comes on more slowly but may last for a longer period of time with more and more follicles becoming involved in resting, which means fewer and fewer follicles producing hair. Triggers for this TE pathway are usually experienced over a prolonged period of time— that is, a persistent cause rather than a one-time event, which could include chronic stress, depression, use of antidepressants, chronic illness, and nutritional deficiencies (e.g., iron, other minerals, vitamins, or amino acid proteins).

3. Hair follicles pass through shorter and shorter growth cycles resulting in thin scalp hair and continuous shedding of the shorter, thinner hairs. Triggers for this TE pathway include on-again, off-again metabolic situations such as chronic stress, crash dieting, and nutritional imbalances; exposure to toxins such as excessive vitamin A or excessive iron supplementation; and hypothyroidism, which can also occur in people being treated for hyperthyroidism. Someone who has already noticed hair loss from androgenetic alopecia may also have concomitant telogen effluvium, with a pattern of shorter and shorter growth cycles. Chronic telogen effluvium also involves shorter growth cycles and short but recurring periods of shedding.

Causes of Telogen Effluvium

Several underlying conditions can result in acute telogen effluvium, including the use of certain drugs, exposure to toxic chemicals, hypothyroidism, iron deficiency, severe illness such as kidney or liver failure, nutritional deficiency or excess (such as a toxic reaction to excess vitamin A, a condition called *hypervitaminosis A*), response to a crash diet (protein malnutrition), sudden changes in hormones either after childbirth (*postpartum*) or after an acute systemic illness with high fever. Acute or chronic stress is considered to be a significant factor in inducing acute telogen effluvium. A stressful event may bring on the condition or generalized stress may aggravate TE when it has been caused by another underlying condition such as any of those listed above. If no significant trauma or stressful events preceded the hair loss, and none of the known causative conditions are present, and hair does not begin to grow back with attempts to correct underlying conditions, physicians may consider *syphilitic alopecia* as the diagnosis—that is, underlying venereal disease may be the cause of hair loss. Because of the existence of so many possible causes, a careful diagnostic evaluation is needed so that effective measures can be taken to correct the underlying condition.

Symptoms of Telogen Effluvium

Noticeable shedding is the prevalent symptom with both chronic and acute TE. Women with idiopathic CTE (i.e., CTE with no known cause) report noticing fairly constant severe shedding of hair for periods of time, but not necessarily *all* the time. Hair can also become generally thinner all over the head, similar to AGA, which can, of course, complicate diagnosing the condition. One differentiating factor is that a receding hairline at the temples may be noticed in chronic or acute TE, although it is not typical of AGA. (Other differentiating factors are described in chapter 4. Hairs on the limbs and pubic area can be affected as well as those on the scalp. Typical losses in acute TE can be about 50 percent of the person's hair; greater losses (70 to 80 percent) may be a sign of serious metabolic disturbances, toxic exposure, or the use of certain drugs. In chronic TE, losses can fluctuate, becoming severe at one time and mild at another.

Treatment for Telogen Effluvium

Effective treatment or management of an underlying condition, either a stress-related condition or an illness such as thyroid disease, is the approach most commonly used to correct telogen effluvium and reverse the shedding. For example, if TE is the result of medication usage, changing the medication or stopping its use is the route to restoring the hair growth cycle. Chronic TE is sometimes treated with a hair growth stimulant such as minoxidil, since this idiopathic form arises on its own with no known underlying cause.

Prognosis for Telogen Effluvium

Acute hair loss resulting from telogen effluvium is usually corrected when the underlying condition is corrected such as discontinuing a specific drug, correcting iron or vitamin deficiency or excess, effectively managing hypothyroidism, or responding well to counseling for underlying stress. Acute TE that has followed childbirth or a severe illness will typically last just a few months and complete recovery will occur on its own when either hormone levels are restored naturally or the individual has recovered from the illness. In idiopathic chronic telogen effluvium, however, hair shedding can last for years; although it may be continuous throughout adult life, the condition can be mild with only minor losses of hair.

HAIR LOSS RELATED TO IRON-DEFICIENCY

Hair loss that develops as a result of iron deficiency is usually a form of acute telogen effluvium and will follow the general characteristics of that disorder as described previously. Iron deficiency is a fairly common mineral deficiency, easy to diagnose with serum ferritin levels, and usually easy enough to treat with some form of iron supplementation. Iron deficiency has long been considered to blame for skin, nail, and hair problems, and the fact that the hair problem is corrected effectively with iron replacement therapy is proof enough that it does cause hair loss—in other words, if reversing the deficiency reverses the hair loss, the diagnosis may indeed be iron deficiency hair loss. Iron deficiency has also been linked with causing androgenetic alopecia and alopecia areata as well as the more common acute telogen effluvium, which typically occurs in conjunction with loss of blood from injury, surgery, or childbirth. Iron deficiency–related hair loss, however, can occur *without* any iron-deficiency anemia or without the loss of any significant amount of blood. In these cases, chronic telogen effluvium or female pattern baldness of androgenetic origin may be considered. A definitive diagnosis may be difficult to obtain.

Causes and Symptoms of Iron Deficiency–Related Hair Loss

The risk of iron deficiency can be increased by loss of blood, consuming large amounts of over-the-counter products containing zinc, drinking large amounts of tea containing tannins and manganese, or taking calcium with meals or with iron supplements. People can also become iron deficient through poor general nutrition. Iron deficiency may first be noticed through symptoms of fatigue or weakness, or hair loss may be noticed first and iron levels tested as a diagnostic measure. If hair loss is diffuse with all-over thinning, either chronic telogen effluvium or late-onset androgenic alopecia may be suspected, perhaps triggered by the iron deficiency. The only real proof will be if reversing the deficiency reverses the hair loss.

Treatment and Prognosis for Iron-Deficiency Alopecia

The only treatment for iron deficiency is iron supplementation. If it corrects the alopecia, it confirms the diagnosis. Levels of other minerals such as zinc, calcium, and manganese should also be evaluated in individuals who are suspected of being iron deficient, because mineral imbalances can be a general metabolic problem that can affect the assimilation of dietary iron. If iron deficiency is confirmed, a long process of treatment for androgenetic alopecia in conjunction with correcting the iron deficiency may eventually reverse the hair loss. Meanwhile, physicians are not all convinced that iron deficiency is a trigger for hair loss, which leaves treatment a case-by-case proposition related not only to iron deficiency but a woman's age, hormonal status, diet, and existing health problems.

HAIR LOSS IN THYROID DISEASE

Hair loss that develops as a result of hypothyroidism, which can occur in people being treated for a range of thyroid conditions, including autoimmune Hashimoto's disease, Graves' disease, or even thyroid cancer, is usually considered to be the third form of telogen effluvium in which hair follicles pass through shorter and shorter growth cycles causing thin scalp hair and continuous shedding of the shorter, thinner hairs. Since autoimmune diseases tend to cluster, individuals with autoimmune alopecia may also have auto-immune thyroid disease, and therefore an association in the medical litera-ture with thyroid disease and alopecia areata, although thyroid disease does not cause this condition. Women with hyperthyroidism (overactive thyroid gland) or thyrotoxicosis (too much circulating thyroid hormone) can experi-ence changes in the nature of their hair, as the hair shafts are finer, but there is not typically thinning of the hair on the scalp. If they are prescribed beta blockers for tachycardia (fast pulse), beta blockers are a class of drug that can cause TE. Additionally, many women who are being treated for hyperthy-roidism may also experience hypothyroidism, which can also result in TE. Women with thyroid disease are well aware of hair shedding, thinning, or the appearance of thinning when hair becomes finer. Physicians and researchers readily acknowledge hair loss as a symptom of thyroid disorders; however, diagnosis of a specific form of alopecia may be difficult, since thyroid disor-ders involve hormone imbalances that can also trigger androgenetic alopecia, another hormone-related condition. The discussion here is about thyroid-related telogen effluvium.

Causes and Symptoms of Hair Loss Related to Thyroid Disease

Hypothyroidism and hyperthyroidism are both characterized by fluctuat-ing thyroid hormones and the resulting hormonal imbalance is sufficient to trigger termination of the anagen phase of the hair growth cycle and a shift toward more and more hairs entering the telogen or resting phase. No scarring or inflammation are present—just increased shedding of the thinner, shorter hairs, with typical losses including from 20 to 50 percent of scalp hairs. Cer-tain medications used to treat hyperthyroidism have also been associated with hair loss because they can cause hypothyroidism (in this case, the hair loss is caused by hypothyroidism and not by the drug), but the only thyroid medi-cations that actually cause hair loss per se are beta blockers, which can also be used for a number of other conditions not related to thyroid disorders. Any treatment that renders the thyroid gland completely inactive, or surgical removal of the thyroid gland that results in permanent hypothyroidism, may result in hair loss if thyroid hormone levels are not restored.

Treatment for Hair Loss Related to Thyroid Disease

Effective treatment of hypothyroidism can correct telogen effluvium and reverse shedding, but it may be difficult or take considerable time to stabilize thyroid hormone balance in some patients. Stimulating hair growth may be an effective approach in some individuals with thyroid-related hair loss and physicians will prescribe a hair growth stimulant such as minoxidil. When a beta blocker appears to be associated with hair loss, it is terminated unless the risks of terminating the beta blocker are greater than the drug side effect of alopecia. There are many thyroid cancer patients who need to be on a higher dose of thyroid hormone, for example, to prevent recurrence, and for them, a beta blocker helps to keep their heart rate stable. Some women decide to live with alopecia if the beta blocker greatly improves their quality of life.

Prognosis for Hair Loss Related to Thyroid Disease

Because telogen effluvium is not a scarring form of alopecia, the hair follicles will remain normal and hair loss can usually be reversed when thyroid hormone levels are restored. If the thyroid gland is rendered inactive or is surgically removed, and the resulting hypothyroidism leads to hair loss, this, too, can be reversed.

LOOSE ANAGEN SYNDROME (ALSO CALLED SHORT ANAGEN SYNDROME)

Somewhere between telogen effluvium, the result of an extended telogen phase, and anagen effluvium, the result of an interruption in the growth phase, is *loose anagen syndrome*, a hair loss condition in which scalp hairs can easily be pulled out with normal combing and brushing. It occurs only in Caucasians and most often in young, fair-haired girls aged 2 to 5 years. It's precise cause is not known although it has been known to occur within families. Because the condition does not typically continue into adulthood, it is not discussed further in this book. It's important to note that loose anagen syndrome can be misdiagnosed as telogen effluvium, alopecia areata, or trichotillomania because symptoms are similar; the reverse can also be true and careful differential diagnosis is required. The syndrome usually reverses spontaneously as the affected child matures and does not require treatment as with other forms of hair loss.

ANAGEN EFFLUVIUM (ALSO CALLED ANAGEN ARREST OR TOXIC ALOPECIA)

Effluvium, as in telogen effluvium, refers to excess flow and "too much telogen," occurring as a result of a disruption in the resting phase of the hair growth cycle. In anagen effluvium, however, it is the anagen or growth phase that is disrupted; *anagen effluvium* essentially means "hair lost during the growth period."

Each of the effluviums affects a different phase of the hair growth cycle—either the two-to-five-year anagen phase in which 80 to 90 percent of hair follicles are producing hair or the two-to-three-month telogen phase in which 10 to 20 percent of hair follicles are resting, producing no growth of hair fiber. In anagen effluvium, which is also called *toxic alopecia*, rather than having an excessive anagen phase of follicular hair growth, the anagen phase is interrupted or "arrested" as a result of a toxic reaction, and hair follicle activity becomes suspended so that hair fibers quickly fall out. The toxic reaction acts as a sudden dramatic shock to the matrix cells of hair follicles. When exposure to toxic substances has damaged the hair matrix, the hair shaft will actually take on a different shape, becoming narrowed or tapered. The hair shaft will then fracture at the narrowest place on the shaft. Some individuals can develop a mix of telogen and anagen effluvium, which can result in complete balding. Individuals who have alopecia areata may also develop anagen effluvium if severe inflammation damages the hair matrix.

We cannot really call anagen effluvium "unexplained" alopecia because it is always caused by toxic reactions and when the causative toxic substance is removed, the hair loss can be reversed. Regardless of the exact cause, anagen effluvium is a nonscarring form of alopecia, which means that the hair follicles remain intact and regrowth is essentially certain.

Causes of Anagen Effluvium or Anagen Arrest

Anagen effluvium occurs most often in individuals who are being treated with cytostatic or cytotoxic drugs for cancer or who have ingested or been exposed to other toxic substances or poisons that interrupt normal cell production. Hair follicle cells reproduce rapidly and can be easily affected by drugs designed to stop or retard cell growth, thereby halting the normal anagen phase in the hair growth cycle. The cytostatic drugs most often responsible for severe, complete hair loss are doxorubicin, a group of drugs called nitrosoureas, and cyclophosphamide, although several other drugs or combinations of drugs can also cause the condition, including:

- Amsacrine
- Cisplatinum
- Cytosine arabinoside
- Epirubicin
- Etoposide
- Ifosfamide
- Vincristine

Chemotherapeutic agents that are not as likely to cause hair loss include:

- Actinomycin
- Bleomycins
- Daunorubicin
- Methotrexate
- Carboplatin
- Mitomycin C
- Vinblastine

Radiation is another major cause of anagen effluvium and dosage is an important factor just as it is in chemotherapy, even though actual dosage to cause hair loss may vary among individuals. Scalp hair follicles are more sensitive to radiation than other areas of the body, but hair follicles in the armpit, beard, eyelashes, and pubic area can also be affected. Hairs that have been exposed to radiation appear tapered when examined microscopically, and the length of the tapered part of the hair varies according to the radiation dose intensity and duration of exposure. Hair loss can occur suddenly after radiation treatments, with large clumps lost almost overnight.

Nonchemotherapeutic drugs, including bismuth, levodopa, and cyclosporine, may also cause anagen arrest. Poisonous chemicals such as boron, thallium, and arsenic can also result in anagen effluvium. The severe inflammation present in alopecia areata can also damage the hair matrix and suspend the anagen phase, resulting in a combination of alopecia areata and anagen effluvium. Endocrine disease and certain types of trauma can also cause anagen effluvium by either damaging the hair matrix or suspending the hair growth phase. A rare type of anagen effluvium stems from a serious autoimmune disease that occurs in middle age, manifesting first as erosive sores in the mouth, which later spread to other parts of the body (*pemphigus vulgaris*). When the sores affect the scalp, the hair matrix can be damaged and hair growth can be suspended.

Symptoms of Anagen Effluvium

Diffuse hair loss is the primary symptom of anagen effluvium; it usually begins and progresses rapidly, resulting in loss of hair from the entire head since the majority of follicles on the scalp are usually in anagen phase. Actual clumps of hair can be found on the individual's pillow during the shedding period.

Treatment for Anagen Effluvium

The only effective treatment for toxic or chemotherapy-related anagen effluvium is removal of the substance that triggered suspension of anagen activity. In European countries, a cold treatment (hypothermia) is used in conjunction with chemotherapy to prevent hair follicles from absorbing the cytotoxic drug, which can reduce the toxic reaction but not prevent hair loss entirely. Application of minoxidil has also been shown to shorten the hair loss period after chemotherapy or radiation, although it does not prevent hair loss. Anagen effluvium that occurs in conjunction with telogen effluvium or alopecia areata will be treated by treating the underlying condition. If it occurs as a result of the autoimmune disease pemphigus vulgaris, treatment will depend on effectively treating the primary autoimmune disease.

Prognosis for Anagen Arrest

Complete reversal of anagen effluvium is to be expected following discontinuance of chemotherapy, removal of the causative drug, radiation, or poisonous chemical, or correcting the condition that is damaging the hair matrix. Hair growth usually resumes within two weeks, almost as rapidly as the onset once the trigger is identified and removed. The rapid result is because follicle activity in anagen effluvium is suspended or "arrested" rather than stopped entirely, and once the offending substance is removed, normal activity simply resumes. Successful treatment of anagen effluvium that is associated with another condition depends on effective treatment of that condition. Because anagen effluvium is a nonscarring form of alopecia, which allows the hair follicles to remain intact, the potential for regrowth is almost certain. New hair growth may be a different color and texture than the individual's original hair. In some cases, the interrupted anagen phase will not resume and hair will not begin to grow until after catagen and the next telogen phase, which will be sometime after one hundred days.

CICATRICIAL ALOPECIA—OR SCARRING ALOPECIA

Cicatricial alopecia is hair loss that is derived from conditions that damage hair follicles and the scalp beneath. Also called *scarring alopecia*, this type of hair loss affects men and woman around the world who are otherwise healthy, most often stemming from an underlying illness of some kind. About 3 percent of all hair loss cases are diagnosed as cicatricial alopecia. Conditions that can lead to cicatricial hair loss include infections (e.g., syphilis, tuberculosis, herpes zoster, or acquired immunodeficiency syndrome, known as AIDS), autoimmune disease, injuries, burns or radiation therapy, dissecting cellulitis, pustular folliculitis, follicular degeneration syndrome (*hot comb* alopecia), and several types of fungi. Regardless of the underlying cause, or even in the absence of a known cause, cicatricial alopecia involves irreversible damage to hair follicles and subsequent development of scar tissue that stops hair growth from any follicles that are damaged. Scarring that has developed over hair follicles will be noticeable when the physician examines the scalp. The doctor will pay special attention to the amount and location of damaged follicles. Biopsy of scalp tissue with microscopic examination will reveal inflammatory cells found in the area around hair follicles. Researchers have suggested that these inflammatory cells are responsible for destroying the follicles and producing the scar tissue. However, because these inflammatory cells are not found in all cases, dermatologists do not all agree that they are the direct cause of scarring alopecia.

Primary cicatricial alopecia is a scarring alopecia in which hair follicles are destroyed, including the opening from which hair fibers usually protrude. No other parts of the body are usually involved and no underlying illness is usually present. When inflammatory cells are found in primary cicatricial alopecia, the condition is categorized further into lymphocytic, neutrophilic, or mixed alopecia, based on the specific type of white cells (leukocytes) that have been found. A type of primary cicatricial alopecia called *keratosis follicularis spinulosa decalvans* affects teenagers. A form called *central centrifugal alopecia* affects African-American individuals more than other races. *Frontal fibrosing alopecia* occurs in postmenopausal women. An auto-immune form of primary cicatricial alopecia, called *chronic cutaneous lupus erythematosus*, may be genetically caused since it develops in individuals whose family has a history of autoimmune diseases. Lupus erythematosus is an auto-immune disease that affects joints and other body organs; it may or may not have been diagnosed in individuals with the alopecia of the same name.

Secondary cicatricial alopecia involves the presence of an underlying illness, which may be a systemic disease affecting other organs of the body and damaging to tissue elsewhere in the body as well as scalp tissue.

Causes and Symptoms of Cicatricial Alopecia

The causes of the various types of primary cicatricial alopecia are unknown. The range of causes for secondary cicatricial alopecia includes radiation to the body, use of certain drugs or exposure to chemicals, surgery, burns, tumor growth, cancer, and autoimmune diseases that involve inflammation of tissue.

Hair loss can be gradual in cicatricial alopecia, and no symptoms at all may show up for a long period of time. Depending on the cause of scarring, the individual may experience severe itching or burning of the scalp, which can be accompanied by pain and all symptoms can progress fairly rapidly. Although not much can be seen on the scalp surface, inflammation can be at work destroying the hair follicles in skin layers below the surface. Signs of inflammation may develop as symptoms progress, including redness and scal-ing. Pigmentation of the skin may change—either increasing and becoming darker, or decreasing and becoming lighter or even white. Some causes of cicatricial alopecia may produce sores that appear as little pustules that drain. Bald patches develop eventually, although toward the end of scarring alope-cia, no further spreading of the bald spots occurs and other symptoms such as burning or itching will also go away. Biopsies taken at this point, however, will not necessarily show that inflammation has also ceased.

Bald patches on the scalp in scarring alopecia no longer have hair follicles. Follicles at the edges of the bald patches, however, may not have been completely destroyed and hair may begin to grow again, reducing the size of the patches. Otherwise, it is not typical to find any regrowth of hair in the patches since scars remain deep in the scalp tissue.

Treatment for Cicatricial Alopecia

After primary or secondary cicatricial alopecia has been diagnosed, the treatment goal will be to control or stop the hair loss as quickly as possible. In secondary cicatricial alopecia, medical care will involve aggressive treatment of the underlying condition that caused cicatricial alopecia.

Prognosis for Cicatricial Alopecia

Cicatricial alopecia, regardless of the cause, does not usually result in the regrowth of hair when follicles have been destroyed in affected areas.

FOLLICULITIS—A FORM OF CICATRICIAL (SCARRING) ALOPECIA

Local inflammation of hair follicles with acnelike eruptions is referred to as folliculitis. Specific types of folliculitis include *eosinophilic pustular folliculitis* and *folliculitis decalvans*, but these and others are essentially the same condition with different underlying causes. Affected follicles will be surrounded by a red ring of inflamed tissue. Hairs will remain intact in the early infection stages but may eventually fall out. If inflammation has been severe or prolonged, follicles can be permanently damaged and bald patches may occur as a result.

Causes and Symptoms of Folliculitis

Folliculitis can be caused by bacterial or viral infection or by a buildup of grease or oils applied to the scalp that clog the hair follicles. Staph infection (*Staphylococcus aureus*) is sometimes the cause of folliculitis. *Pseudomonas aeruginosa*, a type of bacteria that grows in unchlorinated water (such as in hot tubs), can also cause folliculitis; this type is often called *hot tub folliculitis*. Certain viruses, yeasts, and fungi may also cause inflammation of follicles.

Inflammation and acnelike eruptions on the scalp will be noticed. The affected area may feel hot and itchy or irritated. Scarring may develop in severe cases.

Treatment for Folliculitis

Topical application of over-the-counter antibiotic creams (e.g., Bacitracin, Mycitracin, and Neomycin) may be used as well as prescription antibiotics such as Erythromycin or Griseofulvin.

Prognosis for Folliculitis

Folliculitis typically responds to antibiotic treatment and no permanent damage or permanent hair loss may result. However, severe or prolonged inflammation may cause permanent damage to hair follicles, resulting in scarring and eventual permanent hair loss more typical of cicatricial alopecia.

TINEA CAPITIS (TINEA OF THE SCALP) OR RINGWORM

Tinea capitis is a fungal infection that affects the scalp and hair follicles; although it is caused by several different types of fungi, the condition is always called *tinea capitis*. When this type of fungus attacks the skin almost anywhere on the body, it is commonly called ringworm; between the toes it is called athlete's foot, but the scientific name, tinea capitis, is used for scalp infections. On the scalp, tinea capitis typically begins with the presence of a small pimple-type sore that expands into a larger, round scaly sore and eventually causes patches of hair loss and scarring of the scalp. The fungus can get into the hairs themselves, causing hair breakage and, again, bald patches. The fungus can affect anyone but is most common in children and young people between age ten and early teens, causing both ringworm and the scarring scalp condition that eventually results in hair loss. The infection is contagious.

Causes of Tinea Capitis

Several types of fungi can be responsible for causing fungus infections of the scalp. Classic ringworm is caused most often by *Microsporum audouini* in most areas of the world, and *Trichophyton tonsurans* in Latin American countries. Several other fungi can be responsible in other geographic locations, most often affecting humans through contact with the fungus in soil or in animals infected by the fungus. In the United States, even house pets that go outdoors, especially cats, can carry the fungus. People can transfer it to other people through direct contact with an open sore. Contact with contaminated personal items such as combs and brushes, soiled clothing, and bathroom surfaces can also spread the fungus, causing infection in another person. Dampness and warmth create an ideal climate in which fungi can grow. Risk is higher for tinea capitis when hygiene is poor, open skin or scalp injuries are present, or the skin is moist for long periods of time, as from prolonged sweating.

Symptoms of Tinea Capitis

Although tinea capitis may begin with a small, white pimple-type sore, it leads to the formation of round, red, scaly sores that erupt into patches of itching, oozing blisters. Infected patches may be redder around the outside rim, looking rather like a circle or classic ringworm. On the scalp, some infected areas may appear bald because hair has broken off. Small black dots may also be present on the scalp, or pus-filled sores may develop. Itching is not always present.

Treatment for Tinea Capitis

Antifungal medications, either oral or topical, or antibiotic treatment is usually required for tinea capitis infection, depending on the particular fungus responsible for the infection. Griseofulvin has been shown to be an especially effective antibiotic for tinea capitis because it actually blends with the hair fiber and blocks fungi from infecting the keratin in the hair.

Prognosis for Tinea Capitis

Tinea capitis infection can sometimes resolve by itself with no scarring of the scalp. Longer-lasting infections that require antifungal or antibiotic treatments may clear up eventually with effective treatment, but some fungi are resistant and long courses of treatment may be needed, during which the risk of scarring is high. Hair loss is sometimes reversible if scarring of the scalp is minimal with little permanent damage to hair follicles.

TRACTION ALOPECIA—COSMETIC OR TRAUMATIC ALOPECIA

Not precisely a skin condition, traction alopecia is hair loss caused by grooming styles that create high tension and the breaking off of hairs and repetitive hairstyling practices that damage hair follicles. Types of trauma to the scalp that have been known to result in traction alopecia include tight braiding of hair for long periods of time, regularly pulling back the hair tightly to form ponytails, and other tightly woven styles (e.g., cornrows or dreadlocks) worn consistently; use of curling irons, brush rollers, and chemical treatments (e.g., perms, straightening agents, coloring or bleaching products); and use of hairbrushes with square or angled tips. Even the wearing of hats with tight bands around the head can result in traction alopecia if it is done consistently.

Causes and Symptoms of Traction Alopecia

Mechanical action results in traction alopecia. The action is the pulling or "traction" of hair in a repetitive manner that pulls hair out of the skin by its roots and leaves bald patches or areas of thin hair. When the hair is repeatedly pulled into a high-tension hairstyle, hair follicles can become damaged from the repetitive action, and damaged so much that hair growth may be permanently affected.

Treatment and Prognosis for Traction Alopecia

Changing the repetitive hairstyling practice is usually all that is needed to correct traction alopecia unless permanent damage to hair follicles has occurred. Medical treatment is not necessary in the absence of permanent damage to hair follicles. Hair growth will usually be restored when the underlying mechanical trauma is stopped.

PHYSICAL HAIR DAMAGE—OVERPROCESSING OF HAIR AND "BUBBLE HAIR"

Physical hair damage, damage to the hair shaft itself, can occur through combinations of overprocessing of the hair with chemical agents, cuticle stripping, and ultraviolet (UV) light exposure. Damage to the outer cuticle and the inner cortex of the hair can lead to splitting and breakage and, in severe cases, to weakening of the hair fiber at its root. When hairs break off at the skin surface, the result can be diffuse alopecia.

Exactly how does this happen? As we've learned, the tough outer cuticle of the hair shaft is a protective layer of overlapping dead cells. When permanent waves, hair straighteners, bleaches, and coloring chemicals do their work, the cuticle must first be opened to allow the other chemicals access to the cortex of the hair so that the normal chemical bonds of the hair structure can be released. If the chemicals that open the cuticle remain on the hair too long or are applied in high concentration or too often, it can cause permanent cuticle damage, even completely stripping the cuticle away in some cases. The cortex is then directly exposed to environmental damage from detergents in harsh shampoos, chemicals in water or the air, and UV light exposure. Any of these damaging factors can weaken the cortex and cause significant damage to the hair fiber. Fibers can break off at the follicles, causing loss of hair over the entire head in some severe cases—severe diffuse alopecia.

Bubble hair is a condition caused when water gets under the cuticle and into the cortex. The water droplets may then be heated and expanded when the hair is dried on the high setting of a hair dryer. Spaces will develop in the hair fiber and the little bubbles typical of "bubble hair" will form inside the cortex. The bubbles will weaken the hair and cause it to break off, a problem that can become much worse in the presence of hair-processing chemicals.

Treating Damaged Hair or Avoiding Overprocessed Hair

Physical damage to the hair is difficult to treat medically, especially with the addition of more chemicals. Dermatologists advise a gentle approach, first cutting off the damaged hair and then avoiding any additional processing. It is better to wait for undamaged new hair to replace what has been lost than to use cosmetic treatments that promise to restore damaged hair by "gluing" it back together to appear fuller. These cosmetic treatments last only a short time and must be reapplied frequently. Although waiting for a new growth cycle to produce hair may take some time, the resulting hair is usually of normal quality.

TRICHORRHEXIS NODOSA

Trichorrhexis nodosa is a common hair shaft defect—another type of physical defect that can lead to hair breakage over the entire head. Trichorrhexis nodosa can be either present at birth (congenital) or acquired. It involves areas along the hair shaft where no cuticle is present, resulting in very weak hairs. Metabolic disturbances such as abnormal mineral utilization and overprocessing as described above can also result in trichorrhexis nodosa. Excessive brushing or washing, hairstyling that stresses the hair, and overprocessing such as coloring, bleaching, or perming, can also disrupt the cuticle along the hair shaft. When the cuticle is damaged sufficiently, the hair cortex will eventually break down, hairs will break off at the follicle, and hair loss will become apparent.

Treatment for Trichorrhexis Nodosa

Differentiating trichorrhexis nodosa from other types of physical defects may be difficult—first the absence of cuticle along the hair shaft must be identified, and then identification of a possible external cause. If the hair loss condition recurs frequently without the use of chemicals that are known to damage hair, it may indicate a congenital rather than acquired condition and a dermatologist should be consulted before experimenting with cosmetic hair care products. If an external cause is identified such as overprocessing, treatment will be as recommended for other physical damage—cutting off the damaged hair, avoiding any hair-processing procedures, and waiting for undamaged new hair to replace what has been lost rather than using cosmetic treatments to achieve a fuller appearance. As with other types of physical damage that result in hair loss, restoration of normal growth and normal appearance is worth the wait.

TRICHOTILLOMANIA—A BEHAVIORAL PROBLEM THAT RESULTS IN HAIR LOSS

Trichotillomania, or "trich," is a form of hair loss unlike other forms of alopecia because it does not involve hair follicles or the growth cycle. Instead, it involves the compulsive pulling and plucking of one's own hair, a behavioral characteristic (mania) usually associated with a traumatic life event or an ongoing stressful situation. Psychologists prefer to classify the disorder as an impulse control disorder rather than to identify the condition as an obsession or as compulsive behavior. In adults, trichotillomania is more common in women than in men, and although the hair-pulling habit usually develops between the ages of 12 and 29, it may not be diagnosed until signs are seen. The condition actually occurs most commonly in children before age 2, occurring equally among boys and girls. In toddlers the hair-pulling habit and related hair loss are usually milder than in older individuals, although the condition can begin in childhood and continue into adulthood, becoming more progressive if untreated. Trichotillomania usually responds to behavior modification therapy, which helps affected individuals become aware of the hair-pulling habit and then helps them adopt certain techniques to resist the urge to pull their own hair. If counseling or behavioral intervention are not sought, especially for affected children or young people, the condition may progress into adulthood and be considered "normal" for the individual. It is reassuring to know that it can be treated in individuals of any age.

Causes and Symptoms of Trichotillomania

Individuals with trichotillomania will often pluck the hair of the scalp to the extent that bald patches occur. The individual may also pluck eyelashes, eyebrows, public hair, hair on the forearm, or on any other area of the body where hair grows. Most often the hair pulling is done with the fingers but some individuals use tweezers, combs, or brushes as well. Some people do it consciously, with focus and almost ritualistically, but others are so used to doing it that it becomes automatic. People with trichotillomania often fix their attention on gray hairs or curly hairs or hairs of a special texture such as coarse hairs, thinking these hairs are "bad" in some way and must be plucked out. Moods of stress, tension, or boredom can aggravate the habit by providing some kind of comfort or avoidance of the negative feelings. Some doctors consider trichotillomania to be like any other habit such as nail biting, and others feel it is more of a psychological problem. Gene mutations have also been identified as being associated with trichotillomania, but only in some individuals. Clinical studies have also shown that the brain neurochemicals serotonin and dopamine may also be involved in trichotillomania. More studies are needed to confirm the roles that genes or neurochemicals may play. Regardless of the actual cause, most individuals are not usually aware of the hair-plucking habit until a bald spot is noticed, and even then the individual may find it hard to stop the plucking. Signs of the disorder include patchy bald spots, missing eyelashes or eyebrows, playing with or chewing on hairs that have been pulled out. Some affected people also try to eat their hair once it's pulled out, which can be dangerous since hair is not at all digestible. Hair balls can form just as the common hair balls formed by cats who groom themselves by licking their hair. Formation of large, matted hair balls (trichobezoar) can occur, which can result in weight loss, frequent vomiting, intestinal obstruction, and death. Trichophagia, or the eating of hair, can also lead to ulceration of the stomach lining from the presence of constant irritation. Deaths from trichophagia have been reported.

Treatment and Prognosis for Trichotillomania

Trichotillomania has been found to be more effectively treated with psychotherapy than medical treatment, although primary care physicians may follow a typical diagnostic process to identify the cause of the hair loss, even including a biopsy to help determine how the hairs are being damaged.

Once trichotillomania has been diagnosed, the physician will likely refer the individual to a mental health professional to identify the underlying trauma. Cognitive behavior therapy (CBT) has been shown to be effective for treating trichotillomania, and able to reverse the pulling habit through monitoring and training. Medications, including antidepressants, may also be used while therapy is ongoing. Hair growth can be restored when the individual's behavior is corrected, but treatment can be challenging and prolonged.

THE IMPORTANCE OF EARLY DIAGNOSIS OF HAIR LOSS IN WOMEN

Speaking generally, and not of a specific type of condition among those just discussed, diffuse hair loss is the outstanding characteristic of most cases of women losing hair. And fortunately, loss usually comes on gradually, remains relatively mild, and in most cases progresses slowly. Remembering that it's rare for a woman to have scalp areas entirely without hair, the earliest possible attention to any degree of loss is essential. I urge you, even if your hair loss can be disguised with creative styling, don't hide hair loss from your physician because it will only make the problem more difficult to treat when you *do* decide it's time to take action. Since a variety of different medical conditions can cause this diffuse pattern of loss, it is most important to have a thorough investigation by a qualified physician or dermatologist so that the most appropriate treatment can be applied as early as possible. When the condition can be identified along with its underlying causes, hair loss can often be reversed. This is good news. Find out more about the diagnostic process and how to prepare for it in chapter 4.

DIAGNOSING HAIR LOSS: WHAT YOUR DOCTOR NEEDS TO KNOW

How hair loss is diagnosed, how one type of alopecia is differentiated from another (differential diagnosis), what diagnostic tests might be performed, what confirms the diagnosis and how you can trust it, drug categories associated with hair loss

AN ACCURATE DIAGNOSIS LEADS TO APPROPRIATE CARE

The causes of alopecia are many and determining the cause and related permanence of hair loss is what eventually determines the most appropriate treatment. Distinguishing the difference between one form of alopecia and another will take time, testing, and the application of special skills and diagnostic capabilities.

Because more than two hundred diseases and a wide range of medications are known to contribute to hair loss, it's easy to understand why the diagnostic process is so important. It's also easy to understand why various forms of hair loss, especially rare forms, may be difficult to diagnose. Sometimes it can take months or even years to identify the underlying cause and to arrive at an accurate diagnosis, even after consultation with several dermatologists. If a woman visits her doctor because of diffuse generalized hair loss, for example, the process of diagnosing her condition can be confusing because various systemic conditions can lead to overall thinning of the hair or substantial shedding. This makes the woman's history a critical element of diagnosis because of subtle differences in the onset and characteristics of various forms of alopecia, and because doctors know that every patient is subject to androgenetic alopecia, more or less. Once the doctor is armed with a carefully gathered history and has made a thoughtful review of primary symptoms and the results of a physical examination, the diagnosis of diffuse hair loss could be one of the three leading causes of hair loss in women—telogen effluvium, alopecia areata, or androgenetic alopecia. There could also be no single obvious diagnosis, and no certainty about whether the hair loss is permanent or temporary. Without certainty about the cause and degree of permanence, no treatment can be recommended with any assurance of results.

Until recently, few dermatologists have specialized in scalp conditions that lead to hair loss. Fortunately, as awareness of hair loss has grown and millions of men and women have begun to seek help, it has encouraged hair and scalp treatment centers to crop up in larger medical centers around the country (see Resources). Your case could possibly be identified by the first physician you visit—we would all wish for that. On the other hand, you may need to search for a dermatologist who will have specific knowledge of the full range of common and rare types of alopecia.

Not only can diagnosis be a slow process, but the ideal treatment may not always be available, since treatments can be equally slow to be developed. This is because alopecia, which is not a life-threatening condition, attracts few researchers as compared with life-threatening conditions like heart disease and cancer, so the long process of investigation and discovery of treatments, as well as subsequent development of new treatments by pharmaceutical companies, is correspondingly slow. Even if a form of alopecia is quickly and correctly identified, no effective treatment may be available and you may feel you are back to square one. Nevertheless, you must still have patience and trust the diagnostic process and the clinicians who can provide a thorough evaluation of your hair loss problem. It helps to remember that most types of female hair loss can be treated either medically or surgically, once your doctor or a physician hair restoration specialist has made the diagnosis.

To help you prepare for the diagnostic workup that will help identify your condition, the elements of a comprehensive diagnostic investigation of hair loss are described next.

PREPARING FOR YOUR DOCTOR'S VISIT

Diagnosing alopecia in women begins with taking a detailed medical history, starting with the most recent events affecting your health, symptoms you may have besides hair loss, and any upsetting situation, event, or stressful condition that preceded the onset of hair loss. Your doctor will want to know about current or previous illnesses, including childhood illnesses, surgeries, and medical conditions for which you are being treated or have been treated; current and prior medications you've taken; typical diet and any supplements you may be taking; lifestyle habits such as smoking, alcohol consumption, and amount of exercise; and family history of hair loss, if any.

Specifically regarding your hair loss, doctors will want to know when, where, and how you first noticed your hair loss or thinning, how long it has been occurring, and if you have noticed a characteristic pattern such as only on the front or sides of your head, and so forth. Additionally, it will be important to know if your hair breaks off or is being shed from its roots, and if you've noticed any changes such as increases in the amount of shedding or hair thinning. All of these factors are critical in helping your doctor correctly identify what type of hair loss you may have and perhaps be able to suggest likely causes. Your doctor may then order certain types of laboratory tests, such as blood tests, to help confirm the suspected type of hair loss. Additionally, certain diagnostic procedures, such as a biopsy, may have to be done and will be scheduled as needed.

THE DIFFERENCE BETWEEN SHEDDING HAIR AND LOSING HAIR

It may be helpful to know, before you see your doctor or a dermatologist, what shedding is and how your physician will view it. Doctors report that their patients are especially sensitive to the idea of chronic shedding and are very fearful that they may become totally bald at the rate they are losing hair. But, to the doctor, there's a difference between "losing hair" and "shedding." Basically, three terms are used to describe aspects of what we call hair loss: *shedding* is hair coming out by the roots, *breakage* is breaking of the hair shaft above the root, and *thinning* is less hair covering the head generally. If you think you are shedding, before you decide to pack up handfuls of lost hair in a bag to show your doctor how much you are losing, notice whether you are balding or if your hair is thinning. It's quite likely that you are neither balding nor thinning. Instead, shed hair is usually being replaced as it is shed, so actual balding is not a realistic expectation when chronic shedding is the problem. It is more likely an imbalance between periods of growth (anagen) and periods of rest (telogen) and may be either telogen effluvium or anagen effluvium, which both can produce significant shedding. There is typically no underlying cause for chronic shedding of this type. It can last a few months or several years, coming and going, sometimes according to the seasons. It does not typically result in baldness and the growth cycle finally becomes stabilized by itself, leaving the individual with an acceptable head of hair. Losing hair, however, leads to balding because the hair is not being replaced. This is usually a result of androgenetic alopecia, the hereditary type of hair loss.

UNDERSTANDING SCARRING OF THE SCALP

Before a diagnosis is made, you may also benefit from having an understanding of scarring, which occurs in some forms of alopecia. Your doctor will be looking for scarring while performing a physical examination of the scalp and other parts of the body where hair grows. You may remember the topic of scarring as part of the discussion of cicatricial alopecia, the scarring form of alopecia described in chapter 3, which also talked about nonscarring forms of alopecia and how the presence of scarring may influence the types of treatment and the possible outcomes of treatment. To review, "scarring" means, quite simply, that the hair follicle is destroyed by the alopecia and is replaced by scar tissue. Damaged follicles are easy for the doctor to see just by examining your scalp with the naked eye; individual follicles, or follicular units, may also be surrounded by redness (erythema), scaling, or inflammation. If scarring is present, your condition will likely be diagnosed as *cicatricial* alopecia—and cicatricial, as you may remember, means scarring and actually refers to a whole group of rather rare forms of alopecia, not just one type. In each case, it is scarring that differentiates the condition and identifies it as cicatricial alopecia. Other scarring forms of alopecia are folliculitis, hair loss associated with lupus erythematosus, chronic trichotillomania or traction alopecia, and fungus infections such as lichen planopilaris.

By contrast, androgenetic alopecia and telogen effluvium, the two most common forms of alopecia in women, do not usually produce scarring of the scalp. Nonscarring forms of alopecia such as these do not involve follicle damage and follicular units are not able to be seen when the scalp is examined. Other nonscarring forms of alopecia include alopecia areata, acute trichotillomania, drug-induced anagen effluvium, and alopecia related to venereal disease (syphilitic alopecia).

STEP BY STEP—AN ACCURATE DIAGNOSIS OF HAIR LOSS

You will see a simple, step-by-step description of typical steps involved in diagnosing hair loss conditions on page 80. The process that your physician will likely follow to identify the type of alopecia responsible for your hair loss will be somewhat similar to these steps. Diagnosis will start with your medical history—an especially critical part of the diagnostic process, because alopecia can stem from dozens of causes and up to two hundred diseases. As doctors conduct the physical examination and laboratory tests, the range of possibilities becomes narrower, usually allowing a diagnosis to be made, and then the determination of an appropriate course of treatment. You'll notice at the last step, if clinical laboratory tests are all normal—that is, no androgen excess, no iron deficiency, no thyroid disease, and no venereal disease—then additional diagnostic testing may have to be done to help find another possible underlying disease or condition that could be causing your hair to fall out, and/or break off, or the hair growth cycle to be out of balance. Deciding on a course of treatment will then depend on identifying the underlying condition, and understanding that treating that condition appropriately will most likely correct the hair loss. It can be a long period of testing and may require lots of patience on your part, but the reward will be a better outlook, knowing that your treatment will ultimately be more appropriate and more successful.

DIAGNOSING DIFFERENT TYPES OF ALOPECIA IN WOMEN*

To diagnose a specific type of alopecia, your doctor will likely follow a diagnostic workup similar to the one shown here. Additional diagnostic tests will be ordered by your doctor as needed to detect specific underlying conditions or diseases that may have led to scarring or nonscarring forms of alopecia.

Medical History

Family health record

History of illnesses, medications

History of psychological trauma, severe stress or stressful event, or physical trauma (accidents, surgery, childbirth, injury)

Physical Findings

Scarring of the Scalp

Punch biopsy will be done:

1. Negative biopsy results: condition may be hereditary or result of trauma, burns, caustic agents/drugs, or radiation.
2. Positive biopsy results: diagnosis may be systemic disease, fungal, bacterial or parasitic infection, or a form of cancer (tumor or neoplasm).

No Scarring of the Scalp

Diagnostic laboratory testing will be done:

1. Hormone testing to investigate androgen excess, diagnostic for androgenetic alopecia
2. Thyroid function tests to rule out hypothyroidism
3. VDRL (Venereal Disease Research Laboratory) and RPR (rapid plasma regain) tests to rule out venereal disease
4. Complete blood count (CBC) and iron studies (ferritin level) to rule out iron deficiency
5. Antinuclear antibody (ANA) tests to rule out lupus erythematosus
6. Microscopic examination of scalp tissue and culture to identify possible fungal or bacterial infection

Positive Lab Test Results

Additional testing as needed to confirm hypothyroidism, venereal disease, iron deficiency, lupus erythematosus, or infection

Normal Lab Test Result

Diagnosis can be nutritional deficiency, drug-induced anagen arrest, toxicity, protein malnutrition, chronic telogen effluvium, severe stress, traumatic trigger, hereditary condition, autoimmune alopecia. Additional diagnostic tests may be done to identify an underlying condition.

*Adapted from C. C. Thiedke, "Alopecia in Women," American Family Physician 67, no. 5 (2003): 1008.

ADDITIONAL DIAGNOSTIC LABORATORY TESTING TO CONFIRM FEMALE PATTERN AGA

Specific diagnostic laboratory tests for hormone activity may be necessary to further evaluate and diagnose androgenetic alopecia (AGA) when hair loss is diffuse, and to differentiate between female pattern AGA with or without the unwanted hair growth (hirsutism) that is typical of androgen excess in women. Hirsutism can produce thick, dark hairs on the face or chest in a malelike pattern. There are many causes for hirsutism, including ovarian or adrenal tumors and androgen excess, which can occur simultaneously with androgenetic alopecia. Tests and possible diagnostic findings include:

- Dehydroepiandrosterone sulfate (DHEA-S)—this hormone level may be normal or elevated in female pattern AGA, with or without androgen excess.
- Testosterone (T)—normal in female pattern AGA, possible elevation in AGA with hirsutism.
- Testosterone estradiol-binding globulin (TeBG)—normal in female pattern AGA, decreased or normal in AGA with hirsutism
- Androgenic index (T/TeBG Prolactin)—normal in female pattern AGA, elevated in female pattern AGA, and can possibly indicate pituitary gland dysfunction such as the presence of a pituitary tumor called pituitary prolactin-secreting adenoma.

EVALUATING YOUR CURRENT STATE OF HEALTH

When evaluating your health status, your doctor will ask about any recent symptoms or changes in health you may have experienced. The doctor will be looking for symptoms or changes that may signal a possible underlying cause for hair loss, including:

- Recent high fever or severe illness
- Recent surgery
- Previously diagnosed autoimmune disease (rheumatoid arthritis, lupus erythematosus, or polymyalgia, among others)
- Recent pregnancy, childbirth, or onset of menopause
- Symptoms of hormonal disorders such as acne, irregular periods, unwanted hair growth, or voice change
- Recent chemotherapy or radiation
- General dietary considerations and nutritional status
- Recent stressful event or situation, current level of emotional or physical stress
- Psychological disorders such as depression or anxiety

Questions Your Doctor May Ask You about Hair Loss

- When did the hair loss begin—or when did you first notice it?
- Was the hair loss gradual or did it come on suddenly?
- What specific kinds of changes did you see?
- Was your hair thinning or shedding? Falling out or breaking?

- Did you have any sensations of itching, burning, or pain?
- Have you had frequent permanents, straightening, or coloring?
- Do you use hair picks, curlers, hot combs, or rubber bands?
- Have you worn your hair in cornrows, braids, or tightly pulled ponytails?
- Did these symptoms follow any traumatic event that might have upset you?
- What happened specifically that upset you?
- How long after the event did hair loss began?
- Prior to the traumatic event or accident, had you been feeling any physical, mental, or emotional stress before your hair loss began?
- Would you describe your hair as "thinning" or are you shedding "handfuls"?
- How much hair do you see in your comb, on your pillow, or in the sink or shower drain?
- Did either of your parents lose hair or become bald at any point in their lives?
- What about brothers or sisters—did they have any hair loss that you know of?
- How are you feeling about losing your hair? What are your biggest concerns?
- Would you consider or have you looked into surgical or nonsurgical hair replacement?

Questions Your Doctor May Ask about Your Health History

- Have you been treated or are you now being treated for a chronic illness, thyroid disease, autoimmune disease, infection, or cancer?
- What medications have you taken? Do you take any medications now?
- Do you have children? How many pregnancies? Miscarriages?
- Have you ever been treated for hormone imbalances?
- Have you been treated for emotional or psychological problems?
- Have you experienced physical stress or injuries? When? What kind?
- Are you undergoing any emotional stress presently?
- What major or chronic illnesses have your parents or family members had?

YOUR PHYSICAL EXAMINATION

To help your doctor understand your general state of health, a physical examination will be performed, including examining your nose, the inside of your mouth and throat, eyes, and fingernails; palpating the glands in your neck and possibly glands under your arms or in the groin area. Physical examination may also include looking for signs of thyroid gland enlargement in the area in your neck where your thyroid gland sits, at the Adam's apple. These areas are examined in addition to your hair and scalp because certain types of hair loss (e.g., alopecia areata) can be associated with nail abnormalities or certain fungus infections (e.g., lichen planus), lupus erythematosus can produce sores in mouth tissue, and an enlarged thyroid gland can be a sign of a thyroid disorder that could influence hair loss. Your skin will be examined on all areas of your body where hair may be found, to determine the condition and integrity of the skin and hair and to identify any possible clues to scalp hair loss. The doctor will be looking for the types of hair—either fine, thicker terminal hairs or thin velluslike hairs and ends that may be brittle, frayed, or sharp.

Examination of the Scalp, Hair Follicles, and Hair Shaft

Examining the scalp will involve checking for redness (erythema) and the presence of any irritation, inflammation, or scaling of the skin. The doctor will also look for scarring—any signs that follicles have been damaged and then replaced by scars. The pattern of this damage will also be important, as will any condition that may indicate an ongoing irritation or infection of skin or hair follicles. Follicles cannot usually be seen, but if irritated or inflamed, or otherwise affected, they may become visible in the nonscarring type of alopecia. The thickness (density) of the hair will be noted by your doctor as well as how your hair is distributed. The doctor will pay special attention to the location and patterns of hair loss, if these are at all noticeable, as well as the distribution of affected hair follicles, if this can be noticed. Sometimes there is no detectable pattern, depending on the type of hair loss or how long the loss has been occurring. The hair shaft itself will be examined for its size or thickness (diameter or caliber), length, shape (round, flat, or irregular), color (because color can change in some conditions), and how easily a hair will break (fragility).

THE PULL TEST

A simple pull test may be performed to help your doctor determine approximately how many hairs are in the telogen or resting phase of the hair growth cycle. The test is done by grasping a section of your hair equal to about sixty hairs and, while creating a little tension by holding hairs upward from the scalp, pulling them gently but firmly, and noting how many can actually be pulled out. If your doctor can remove only six or fewer hairs, it indicates a negative test; if more than six hairs can be removed by pulling, it will indicate a positive test. It's best to perform the test in several locations around the head. This manual test can be definitive for a specific type of alopecia because healthy hair will not come out with pulling. In hair loss characterized as telogen effluvium, for example, a larger percentage of hairs (up to 50 percent) may be pulled out with a pull test. A positive pull test can therefore be diagnostic for telogen effluvium, indicating that up to 50 percent of the hairs are in telogen phase rather than the usual 15 percent. This will vary among individuals, especially in advanced disease. Shampooing or vigorous brushing can affect the pull test by removing a significant number of telogen hairs before the test is performed, causing a negative result that can actually be incorrect (false negative). To avoid this, before deciding to do the pull test, your doctor may ask when you last washed or brushed your hair.

When the pull test is done, the pulled hairs are often examined microscopically as well to determine whether there are more hairs in telogen or in anagen phases, and if a fungus infection is present. The root ends of telogen hairs appear swollen, club shaped, and white (almost like a Q-tip) under the microscope. An anagen hair has visible pigment at the root and pieces of the root sheath, which creates a shiny bulblike appearance. Under the microscope, fungus can be seen as tiny spores inside the hair shaft.

PARTING THE HAIR

To help determine the type of alopecia you may have, one of the first things your doctor may do is to make a part in the middle of your scalp from the crown (coronal area) to the front hairline (frontal area). The width of the part will be measured at various points and the results recorded. Results may be compared to widths of smaller diagonal parts made at other locations on the scalp—almost in a Christmas-tree pattern in which the center part is the tree trunk. If the doctor finds that the coronal part is markedly wider than other parts, with no sign of a receding frontal hairline, it is likely that your hair loss is caused by androgenetic alopecia, which quite typically produces this pattern. Besides allowing comparison of part widths in different locations, parting also allows the physician to help evaluate hair density at different parts of the head.

WHAT TO EXPECT IF YOUR DOCTOR ORDERS A PUNCH BIOPSY

Scalp biopsy is not ordered routinely but may be reserved as another option if the history and physical examination are not able to provide obvious clues to the source of your hair loss. Sometimes, however, especially if any unusual abnormality or scarring of the scalp is present, a punch biopsy will be performed early in the diagnostic process.

The punch biopsy is a way to extract and test a portion of skin from the scalp (tissue specimen) and to identify the actual condition of the follicles and the hair shaft in the portion removed, as well as the presence of inflammation or noticeable changes in the cells of the tissue (fibrosis) and any other noticeable changes in the skin layers of the scalp (dermis and epidermis) that could point to a cause of ongoing hair loss. A punch biopsy is performed using a special needle that is able to extract a piece of tissue from the scalp. This is followed by a special clinical laboratory process that can identify cell types in the scalp tissue or degree of follicle damage that may be indicative of certain types of hair loss.

Your doctor may perform or order a punch biopsy to confirm your diagnosis or to gather useful information about your condition to help diagnose your condition. You should understand up front that it does involve a needle-stick in one or more parts of the scalp, but the procedure is performed under local anesthetic and does not usually produce more than minor discomfort at the site of puncture following the procedure. As with any procedure that breaks the skin, however, complications can and do occur occasionally in some individuals. Complications may include bleeding at the site; pain; infection; allergic reaction to the anesthesia used; or damage to an underlying vein, artery, or nerve in the scalp tissue. Of course, your physician will be especially careful during the procedure and take appropriate precautions to avoid any complications.

The Punch Biopsy Procedure

A pencil-like punch biopsy needle employs a plunger mechanism within it, almost like a syringe, to cut the skin and pull out a cylindrical section of tissue that looks like a little plug or cork. The punch needle looks too small to remove a significant portion of skin tissue, but it's important to remember that the examination involves microscopic viewing of the tissue, which magnifies follicles and hairs significantly. You cannot imagine the difference in actual appearance by the naked eye and a magnified view if you haven't seen it yourself. To refresh the image, go back to chapter 2 and take a look at the drawing of a hair as it would be seen under the microscope.

First, the portion of the scalp to be tested is injected with local anesthesia, numbing these areas so that removal of the biopsy samples cannot be felt. Samples are withdrawn with the needle from several different points on the head—some that you may have reported as being affected and possibly some that are not noticeably affected. When the sample is obtained, it is placed in a sterile container to be sent to the clinical laboratory where it will be imbedded in liquid paraffin, allowed to solidify, and then sliced and stained to be examined microscopically. The microscopic examination is performed in the pathology or histology laboratory by a clinical pathologist who can identify the type of cells in the cross-section of stained sample.

After the biopsy procedure, the injection sites will be closed by stitches (sutured) across the tiny openings and an antibiotic cream will be applied to the skin surface around each incision site. You may be asked to continue using this cream and the doctor may advise other measures to help heal the incisions. You will also be asked to return in a week or two to have the stitches removed. Healing takes place within that time and small scars may form over the biopsy sites. Results of the pathology examination should be available at the time your stitches are removed. Results will help your doctor determine treatment for your hair loss problem.

DIFFERENTIAL DIAGNOSIS—USING A PHYSICAL EXAM AND TESTS TO IDENTIFY TYPES OF ALOPECIA

Differential diagnosis involves weighing all of the diagnostic criteria—the history, symptoms, physical examination, and the results of laboratory tests and diagnostic procedures—to identify differences among the various forms of alopecia and to determine which form is affecting the individual patient.

It requires comprehensive knowledge of all forms of alopecia and as much information as possible about the patient and her hair loss condition. Visual signs observed by your physician during the physical examination will help greatly with differential diagnosis.

Differential diagnosis may also involve identifying a scalp condition or a disease that is affecting hair growth, or appears to be. Diagnostic information may point toward one form of alopecia or several, which may involve more testing to distinguish between possible conditions. Remember, alopecia means balding—balding from any cause. However, if a disease is found to be causing alopecia, treating the disease will be critical in treating the associated hair loss. And if a scalp condition is causing alopecia, the scalp condition must be treated. An accurate diagnosis is the beginning of appropriate treatment for the alopecia. And determining the diagnosis relies as much on ruling out possible alternative causes as identifying the actual cause. It can be a long, complicated process of weeding through details about your case.

Some of the diseases or conditions that your physician is likely to consider or try to rule out may include:

Forms of alopecia—alopecia areata, alopecia mucinosa, androgenetic alopecia, anagen effluvium, cicatricial alopecia, telogen effluvium, traction alopecia, and trichotillomania

Scalp conditions—atopic dermatitis (eczema), pemphigus vulgaris, psoriasis, tinea capitis, and widespread skin disease

Underlying diseases—collagen disease, autoimmune diseases, diabetes mellitus, endocrine (glandular) disorders, hypothyroidism, hyperthyroidism, hypopituitarism, infections, iron deficiency, lymphoma, metabolic disorders, protein malnutrition, and venereal disease (syphilis)

GROUPING THE VARIOUS FORMS OF ALOPECIA

While evaluating your hair loss condition, your doctor has to consider the full range of forms of alopecia and begin to narrow your condition into a category that has similar characteristics. The list on the following page places the major forms of alopecia into logical groupings.

MAJOR FORMS OF ALOPECIA

Diffuse or "All-Over" Hair Loss (Nonscarring Forms)
Androgenetic alopecia
Alopecia areata
Anagen effluvium (chemotherapy, radiation, toxic reaction)
Hair shaft abnormalities
Venereal disease (syphilis)
Telogen effluvium (thyroid disorders, postpartum, postmenopausal, drug-induced, iron-deficiency, malnutrition, physiological, or psychological stress)

Focal or "Spotty" Hair Loss (Nonscarring Forms)
Androgenetic alopecia
Alopecia areata
Trichotillomania
Traction alopecia
Hair shaft abnormalities
Tinea capitis
Venereal disease (syphilis)

Scarring Forms
Injuries/wounds/lacerations
Postsurgical
Burns
Radiation
Tumors (neoplasms)
Discoid lupus erythematosus
Lichen planopilaris
Bacterial infection
Herpes infection

DIFFERENTIAL CRITERIA THAT MAY HELP MAKE A DIAGNOSIS

- *Identifying the source or type of scarring alopecia* (e.g., folliculitis, dissecting cellulitis, follicular degeneration syndrome, and infectious causes) may be difficult if just observing the pattern of hair loss and visual appearance of the scalp skin. A punch biopsy and microscopic examination will usually be needed to see evidence of hair follicle destruction, such as the presence of scar tissue in deeper layers of skin, and the location of inflammation in relation to follicles such as the ring of inflammation around follicles in folliculitis, one form of scarring alopecia.

- *Distinguishing anagen effluvium from telogen effluvium* requires a pull test; hairs removed are examined to compare the number of anagen (growth phase) hairs to telogen (resting phase) hairs; hairs may be examined by light microscopy to determine the difference, although sometimes the difference can be observed with the naked eye. Anagen hairs are fully pigmented with long roots that are covered with sheaths. Telogen hairs are partially depigmented and have short roots shaped like a club; there are no root sheaths.

- *Distinguishing anagen effluvium from other forms of alopecia* may require a punch biopsy with at least 25 to 50 hairs. Fewer than 15 percent of follicles are usually in the telogen phase, so having a normal ratio of anagen to telogen hairs would suggest anagen effluvium; whereas having more than 15 percent of follicles in telogen suggests telogen effluvium. If follicles have no sign of inflammation or trac-tion (evidence of pulling or stretching), anagen effluvium is suggested rather than alopecia areata, androgenetic alopecia, or traction alopecia.

- *Differentiating TE from AGA*: Researchers are exploring ways to differentiate TE from AGA through clinical and diagnostic criteria representative of each type of hair loss. David Whiting, a Dallas dermatologist, conducted research (Whiting, 1995) to establish criteria that would help distinguish between idiopathic chronic telogen effluvium (CTE), so common in women in their 40s, 50s, and 60s, and androgenetic alopecia, which also starts in women around age 50. Dr. Whiting's results indicated that the punch biopsy provided useful information to help distinguish telogen effluvium from androgenetic alopecia, but not without performing additional tests as well. The Whiting study concluded that CTE affecting women between the ages of 30 and 60 usually starts abruptly without a single recognizable cause. CTE can be distinguished from androgenic alopecia (AGA) through different clinical findings (e.g., its long course with hair loss starting and stopping, compared to continuous overall thinning in AGA) and greater numbers of telogen hairs found on punch biopsy. Also, many miniaturized hairs are found in AGA but none at all in CTE. Additionally, a wide center part is common in AGA but uncommon in CTE and a pull test will usually be positive all over the head in CTE but will only be positive on the top of the head in AGA, if at all. Telogen effluvium is suggested if physical stress has been experienced recently such as surgery, pregnancy, or malnutrition, as well as exposure to medications or presence of a serious illness within recent months.

- *Differentiating anagen effluvium from female androgenetic alopecia (AGA)* can be done by comparing the diffuse or all-over hair loss of anagen effluvium from the thinning of hair on the top and sides of the head as in androgenetic alopecia. Presence of redness (erythema), scaling, pustules, or covering of follicle openings may indicate local disease rather than anagen effluvium or another cause besides chemotherapy. Pemphigus vulgaris should be suspected if sores in the mouth are present or are present elsewhere on the body corresponding to sores on the scalp.

- *Drug-induced hair loss must* be suspected in women who are taking any of a variety of medications known to include hair loss as a side effect. Losing hair as a result of taking medications is related to exposing the hair matrix to the toxic effects of the particular drug. Not all medications cause this, of course, and hair loss has only been proven to be associated with a few drug categories—in particular, immunosuppressant or cytostatic (chemotherapy) drugs. How an individual responds to taking a drug depends on the way the medication is absorbed in the body (drug mechanism), the dosage prescribed, and the genetic susceptibility of the individual. As discussed earlier, severe forms of alopecia can be caused by the chemotherapy drugs doxorubicin, nitrosoureas, and cyclophasph-amide; also, but less often, the causative drug could be bleomycin, dactinomycin, fluorouracil, or methotrexate, which are known to produce mild to moderate hair losses in some people. Other causative medications include bismuth, levodopa, and cyclosporine. When a drug is suspected as the cause of telogen effluvium or anagen efflu-vium, the diagnosing physician must also rule out other diseases or scalp conditions by physically examining the hair and scalp, which could reveal another cause besides the suspected drug. The doctor may also stop or change the medication to see if the hair loss condition begins to correct, confirming the drug-related cause. This form of hair loss is not like other alopecias because it is temporary, nonscarring, and because removal of the cause always restores growth.

- *Iron deficiency as a possible trigger for hair loss* can confuse attempts to distinguish between androgenetic alopecia in women and chronic telogen effluvium, since the characteristics of these conditions already overlap to some degree. Each of these conditions involves a high level of hairs in the telogen phase and an overall decrease in hair density, which is seen as diffuse losses of scalp hair. Iron deficiency can develop in women with chronic telogen effluvium without any signif-icant loss of blood or without the presence of anemia. Although iron deficiency may likely be suspected as a factor in hair loss if it occurs following loss of blood from injury, surgery, or childbirth, in other cases, depending on the woman's age and hormone status, androge-netic alopecia will probably be considered first. With women and iron deficiency, the doctor will consider age, hormone status, pregnancy, diet, oral contraceptive use, and either medical problems or possible medications that could cause hair loss. Iron deficiency will probably be addressed by ordering a serum ferritin test, but it will not likely be considered as the primary cause of the hair loss. Although deficiency of the essential nutrients zinc and biotin have been shown to cause chronic telogen effluvium, one article in the *Journal of the American Academy of Dermatology* (Olsen, 2006) has stated clearly that "the jury is still out" on iron deficiency and hair loss. Essentially, if iron supplementation reverses the hair loss, it confirms the diagnosis. It does not mean, however, that androgenetic alopecia or chronic telogen effluvium are not also present, so further testing will be required to differentiate.

- *Tinea capitis* can be positively identified with tests for the causative fungus, but the appearance of the scalp itself is sometimes enough to be sure of the diagnosis. Round, scaly sores will be seen that can be red and swollen, or pus-filled and oozing liquid (kerions). Little black spots may also be seen. The sores occur noticeably in rings with infection concentrated at the outer edges. A biopsy can be done of an infected area and microscopic examination of the sample will show moldlike fungi called dermatophytes. Because the appearance of the scalp is so distinctive, a biopsy is often not needed. Cultures offer another way to identify fungus if appearance is not conclusive. Also, a test called the Wood's Lamp Test may be done to confirm that the infection is caused by a fungus, which then may be identified by biopsy or culture. The Wood's Lamp Test shines ultraviolet light on the infected area while you sit in a darkened room. The examiner holds the lamp about five inches from the infected part of the scalp and looks for color changes in the ultraviolet rays. Normal healthy skin will not fluoresce under the ultraviolet light, but fungus infections will give off a fluorescent glow. The test can give a false negative if the room is not dark enough or if you have recently washed your hair and scalp. Under the right conditions, however, the Wood's Lamp Test can help identify bacterial and fungal infections as well as other conditions (e.g., porphyria and pigmentary alterations).

- *Psychological disorders* such as anxiety, obsessive/compulsive behavior, or impulse disorders, when observed, may suggest trichotillomania even if significant hair loss is not seen.

- *Systemic, chronic illnesses* such as an autoimmune disease or cancer may suggest that the hair loss diagnosis is alopecia areata (autoimmune alopecia) or telogen effluvium.

DRUGS AND DRUG CATEGORIES THAT ARE REPORTED TO CAUSE HAIR LOSS

The effects of drugs on hair are limitless, including graying, darkening, straightening, or curling hair. Drugs can also cause hair loss, hair shedding, or increased growth of hair. Drug-induced hair loss is almost always because of the drug's toxic effect on the hair matrix. The type of alopecia that results is usually either telogen effluvium or anagen effluvium (anagen arrest), or sometimes both forms, either of which can usually be reversed by stopping intake of the drug . (See "Telogen Effluvium" and "Anagen Effluvium," chapter 3.) Androgenetic alopecia may be produced by hormone-related drugs such as estrogen-replacement drugs or oral contraceptives. And a drug called Busulfan, which is prescribed for bone marrow transplantation or brain tumor radiation, can cause scarring alopecia that cannot usually be reversed. Whether taking a drug produces hair loss will depend on the chemical component of the drug, the dosage prescribed, and the susceptibility of the individual receiving it.

Hair loss as a result of drugs will be considered by your doctor in the diagnostic process and, besides reporting any drugs you are taking at the time of your examination, you may need to remember other drugs that have been prescribed for you in the past. For the doctor, it will be a matter of identifying which particular medication is affecting your hair growth or altering your hair growth cycle. All drugs taken until the onset of hair loss will be considered, even though it may be difficult to prove whether or not the drug was the cause of your hair loss. Although only a few drugs have been scientifically proven to cause hair loss, including chemotherapeutic agents, the drugs on the following list, among others, have all been reported to produce hair loss. Many more are implicated:

- Analgesic pain relievers (ibuprofen, indomethacin, naproxen sodium)
- Androgens (oral contraceptives)
- Antidepressants (tricyclic drugs, serotonin uptake inhibitors, fluoxetine)
- Antiepileptics
- Antipsychotics
- Appetite suppressants
- Bismuth

- Blood pressure medications (ACE inhibitors, beta blockers—also used to treat symptoms of hyperthyroidism or thyrotoxicosis)
- Busulfan (used in bone marrow transplantation)
- Chemotherapy agents (doxorubicin, nitrosoureas, cyclophosphamide, bleomycin, dactinomycin, fluorouracil, methotrexate)
- Chloramphenicol
- Cimetidine
- Clonazepam
- Cyclosporine
- Danazol
- Estrogen
- Gentamicin
- Hypocholesterolemic drugs (clofibrate, fenofibrate)
- Immunoglobulins
- Immunosuppressants (leflunomide, methotrexate, mycophenolate mofetil)
- Interferons
- Leflunomide (immunosuppressant)
- Levodopa (prescribed for Parkinson's disease)
- Lithium
- Methotrexate (immunosuppressant)
- Methyldopa
- Minoxidil (a hair growth drug)
- Oral contraceptives
- Radiation
- Retinol (vitamin A)
- Retinoids (acitretin, isotretinoin)
- Salicylates
- Tamoxifen
- Thyroxine
- Vasopressin

Now that you understand more about the steps involved in diagnosing your hair loss condition, you may be ready to jump into that process and let your primary care physician or a dermatologist, or both, start to investigate what's behind the hair loss you've noticed.

And once the diagnostic process gets under way, you will undoubtedly have some questions of your own. Next, you'll find questions that other hair loss patients have had. Your doctor may not yet have the answers, but voicing the questions will help make sure each issue of personal concern is looked into thoroughly.

Questions You May Wish to Ask Your Doctor About Hair Loss

- What type of hair loss do I have?
- What caused my condition?
- Can my type of hair loss be treated? What type of treatment is typical for this type of hair loss?
- Will my hair start growing again? How soon will my hair grow back after I begin treatment?
- How many patients have you seen who now have or previously had hair loss?
- How many or what percentage of your hair loss patients have regrown their hair successfully?
- Among patients whose hair loss conditions did not respond to treatment, what cosmetic solutions were the most popular? Which were the most successful?
- Should I avoid certain hair remedies that are advertised? Specifically, what kinds or brands should I avoid? Can you recommend specific brands to consider?
- Other than professional medical treatment, is there anything I can do for myself to prevent further hair loss or to encourage hair growth?
- What nutrients are known to help hair grow or prevent further loss?
- What type of diet should I follow to get nutrients that may support hair growth?
- While I'm improving my condition and appearance, is there some kind of advice or counseling that will help me restore my sense of confidence and self-worth?
- Can you recommend an appropriate therapist or counselor?

CHAPTER 5

MEDICAL TREATMENTS FOR HAIR LOSS

What's involved in medical treatment, common pharmaceutical therapies for specific types of alopecia, herbal therapies supportive of hair growth, ongoing research for future hair loss treatment, stress reduction as treatment for hair loss

WHAT ABOUT "CURES" FOR HAIR LOSS?

Hair loss is not new so, of course, there's nothing new about seeking "cures" for hair loss. Solutions to the hair loss problem, both cures and camouflages, have been recommended throughout history—some have worked and some haven't. These so-called cures have come from philosophers, early medicine men, witches, sorcerers, and herbalists, with a range of dietary and topical recommendations from bird droppings to bee pollen. Camouflages were just as far reaching and inventive. The wreaths of woven leaves seen on the head of Julius Caesar were supposedly designed to cover his thinning hair. In seventeenth century England, the sixty-five-year-old Queen Elizabeth was described to have "suffered the loss of her hair and her teeth, and in the last few years of her life ... refused to have a mirror in any of her rooms." She has been pictured in elaborate head cover-ups and high collars. In the French court of Louis XIV, both men and women competed for attention by showing off ornate wigs; Louis himself was reported to have invented the style as a cover-up. Similarly, in the most recent movie about France's fashion setter, Marie Antoinette, the same amazing wedding-cake curls and upsweeps appeared on the heads of Marie and her bevy of attendants. Imagine how many of these towering wigs might have covered thinning or balding heads.

If we uncover the cover-up stories, we find that hair loss seems to be an open opportunity for inventiveness to emerge. One of the biggest problems of treating hair loss is, in fact, that hundreds of large and small companies, hair clinics, and even individuals have made an array of products available that claim either to treat or correct thinning hair and overall hair loss, or even more boldly, claim to miraculously regrow new hair. Some of the hair products are applied to the scalp, some are explained as medications or supplements to the diet, some are devices or procedures—and not all have scientific evidence that they achieve the claims made about them. They are also not aimed at the specific types of hair loss among the different forms of alopecia. Some seem to be aimed generally at any type of hair loss, even if it's temporary and reversible. Clearly, as we have learned, some types of hair loss reverse spontaneously, others require treatment of an underlying condition, and still others are allowed to proceed on course because it's understood that the hair growth cycle will eventually normalize.

Meanwhile, other types of hair loss—particularly the most common form, androgenetic alopecia, which can affect the whole head with thinning, patchy balding, or pattern balding—will require treatment to either stop the loss of hair or promote new growth, or both. Medical treatments available for various categories of hair loss are described next, including a discussion of treating stress as a cause or an aggravating factor in hair loss.

DRUG THERAPY FOR FEMALE ANDROGENETIC ALOPECIA

The standard treatment for androgenetic alopecia in men and women focuses on reducing androgen activity, specifically by decreasing levels of dihydrotestosterone (DHT), the androgen whose excess or effects such as miniaturizing hair follicles may result in alopecia. In men, AGA or male pattern baldness is reported to respond favorably to the use of anti-androgen therapies. In women, however, AGA does not develop in exactly the same way and DHT or excess androgens seem to have less influence on development of the condition. Female AGA is characterized by thinning scalp hair in the midfrontal scalp with no changes in the hairline across the forehead. Studies of the use of anti-androgen therapy in women have shown that female AGA does not respond well, and in some women does not respond at all, to the same anti-androgen medications that work for male pattern baldness.

One strategy employed by some physicians who are treating female patients for hair loss is to identify if a woman who reports hair loss or hair thinning may be particularly sensitive to androgens, and try to balance her unbalanced hormones. This is not done by directly reducing DHT, as with any of the drugs currently being used to treat male pattern baldness. Consider that women who are in menopause, or are postmenopausal, are often being treated for symptoms such as hot flashes with hormone replacement therapy, either with estrogen alone or an estrogen-progesterone combination.

Some women may be using a natural source of estrogen replacement such as a hormone cream or lotion applied to the skin. These estrogen replacement regimens work well for some women, but not all, especially not the women who are converting estrogen to androgens that, in turn, have a strong effect on their hair follicles and may produce greater thinning of the hair and other symptoms of androgen excess such as oily skin and acne. Without even performing hormone studies, these women appear to be genetically predisposed to have greater follicle sensitivity to androgens. If they are already on estrogen replacement therapy, their dosage may be adjusted, or they may be switched to oral hormone treatment or to an estrogen-progesterone source. Because transdermal hormones are delivered through the skin right into the bloodstream, they often produce higher levels of hormones at lower doses than when hormones are delivered orally. The point is to reduce the amount of estrogen that is available to be converted into androgens, thereby halting hair loss to some extent. Taking a soy supplement with a good supply of phytoestrogens may also help curb hot flashes sufficiently to allow reductions in oral estrogen (Northrup, 2003). Again, this reduces the amount of estrogen available to be converted to androgens since any estrogen replacement therapy that leads to too much androgen may lead to hair loss. Please understand that it's not that the estrogen replacement regimen itself causes hair loss; rather, it's the imbalance in the body's own hormone production that creates the problem.

Besides hormone imbalances, another factor that may contribute to excess production of androgen is a high-carbohydrate diet—that is, consuming too many foods that have a high glycemic index (foods that boost circulating glucose levels), which can result in producing too much insulin. Eating a diet that lowers insulin production can help avoid excess androgen production. Dr. Christiane Northrup, in her book *The Wisdom of Menopause*, outlines a hormone-balancing food plan that is aimed at restoring balance to insulin and estrogen production. She advocates specific food choices that can deliver multiple benefits, including sleeping better, losing excess fat, reducing the risk of developing the diseases of aging, and producing healthy skin that "takes on a healthy glow" (Northrup, 2003).

Meanwhile, some of the same drugs prescribed for men who wish to correct their male pattern baldness are prescribed for women with noticeable female AGA. Drugs available include minoxidil (Rogaine) and finasteride

(Propecia) although finasteride has not been proven safe or effective in women and has therefore not been approved by the Federal Drug Administration (FDA) for use in women. Minoxidil is considered safe and effective for both men and women; 2 percent and 5 percent solutions are available without prescription as a topical treatment that's applied directly to the scalp. The American Academy of Dermatology includes minoxidil in its guidelines for treating androgenetic alopecia. While using minoxidil, women may be treated simultaneously with estrogen replacement therapy, oral contraceptives, or spironolactone (Aldactone) to help balance the hormonal influences. (Note: Aldactone is a registered trademark of the Upjohn Company.) Treating hair loss with minoxidil may help regrow hair, but if inflammation of the follicles occurs during the course of androgenetic alopecia and actually damages the follicles, miniaturized follicles will not likely convert back to thicker, larger hairs (terminal hairs). This reminds us that loss of hair may be stopped while using a hair growth drug, but it will persist if the drug treatment is stopped. It's also important to note that the use of minoxidil can help enlarge hairs that are still growing and retard general thinning of hair, but is of little benefit for areas of the scalp that are already bald. Clearly, this is of greatest benefit to women who are not seeing significant balding from androgenetic alopecia. Hairs can often be thickened sufficiently to allow hairstyling that can effectively mask the areas of sparse growth. However, it also means that treatment must continue indefinitely to enjoy continued thickening.

The anti-androgen therapies are described next as part of overall AGA management options. Remember that only topical minoxidil is approved for use in women. The other drugs discussed here are approved for use in men with hair loss and are not currently approved for use in women; I discuss them here because, in time, modified formulations may become available for treatment in women.

About Minoxidil

Minoxidil (Rogaine) is sold as a topical solution, a reformulation of a drug that was originally developed by the Upjohn Company as an oral medication for treating high blood pressure (hypertension). Because it was discovered to also result in hair growth in individuals who took it for high blood pressure, it was investigated in clinical trials as a topical solution for the treatment of male pattern baldness. It was later approved by the FDA for the purpose of growing hair, meaning that the drug had been proven in clinical trials to be safe and effective for that specific indication. Additionally, since androgenetic alopecia affects both men and women, the solution was tested in males and females and was approved for use in both genders. Originally introduced as a prescription hair growth medication, minoxidil is now available over the counter in drugstores as either a 2 percent or 5 percent topical solution. A few generic brands are also available for the 2 percent solution of minoxidil. The usual recommended dosage is to apply 1 ml of either recommended solution to a dry scalp twice each day with the applicator provided in packaging, spreading it across the balding area with the fingers. Wetting the head should be avoided for a couple of hours for best results. The 5 percent solution is most often recommended for women even though studies have not shown much difference in results with the stronger solution.

Minoxidil is believed to work by increasing the amount of time that hair follicles stay in the anagen phase of the hair growth cycle. It also encourages growth of the follicles that are in telogen phase, the resting part of the hair growth cycle, and enlarges miniaturized follicles. Significant growth of hair long enough to be combed or styled is seen within eight months in about one third of people using the product twice a day, every day, as recommended. Although the medication has been found to do what it is intended to do, there is some disappointment among the other two thirds of users in the quality of new growth. Growth is not usually as good as desired and hair growth will cease about two to three months after the medication is no longer used or not used as recommended. People using the topical solution must use it consistently and almost for the rest of their life, or for as long as they wish to maintain some level of hair growth and replacement. Many individuals are willing to do so rather than continue to experience progressive baldness or, in women, overall thinning of their hair. Although scalp irritation, itching, redness, and dryness are reported by users as a response to the alcohol and propylene glycol used as a base for the minoxidil, these side effects are not as troubling as possible dizziness from significant decreases in blood pressure. (Remember, minoxidil was originally intended as a blood pressure medication.) If you are thinking about trying minoxidil, be sure to discuss it with your physician first, who will know if you are likely to experience blood pressure problems when using the medication.

About Finasteride

Finasteride (Propecia) was approved by the FDA as an oral therapy for treating androgenetic alopecia in men with male pattern baldness. It is available in 1 mg and 5 mg tablets. Doctors often prescribe the 5 mg tablet and advise their patients to split it into four quarters to significantly reduce the cost of using the drug regularly. The drug is not approved for use in women but is discussed here because there is some interest in a formulation of the drug that may eventually work for women.

The way finasteride works is to block the enzyme (5-reductase type II) that stops conversion of testosterone to dihydrotestosterone (DHT) in the scalp, which is considered to be a cause of the miniaturization of scalp hair follicles characteristic of androgenetic alopecia in men or male pattern hair loss. In clinical trials with male subjects, finasteride was shown to slow the progress of hair loss and to begin to produce new growth within three months of beginning treatment. No change in hair growth cycles was seen in about one third of the men who participated in the clinical trials. Long-term follow-up showed that continuous use is required as with minoxidil. A small percentage of men who have taken finasteride have reported sexual dysfunction as a side effect. Sexual function was restored in these men either by discontinuing the drug or by spontaneous reversal of the problem after continued use. No other side effects were reported in men aged forty or younger.

When the effects of finasteride were studied by Merck scientists in women with female AGA, postmenopausal women who took 1 mg of finasteride a day for one year showed no reductions in thinning of hair and no increase in hair growth. The study was discontinued at that point. One explanation for the failure of finasteride to show significant positive effects on hair growth in this group of study subjects is that the hair loss of postmenopausal women is likely influenced more by the enzyme aromatase than by DHT. Scientists know that finasteride affects DHT levels but does not act on aromatase at all, so this explanation is not only justified, it could preclude any further attempts to study finasteride in women. Postmenopausal women are also known to have fairly low levels of DHT compared with men—another possible explanation for the poor response to finasteride. Although finasteride helps reduce excess growth of hair (hirsutism) in women who have significant androgen excess, it is not recommended for use in women who are pregnant or of child-bearing age because male fetuses could become feminized. Finasteride has therefore not been approved for use in women for hair loss associated with androgenetic alopecia.

About Spironolactone

Spironolactone (Aldactone) was originally developed as a treatment for high blood pressure (hypertension). It works as a diuretic, reducing the amount of fluid excreted by the body, which also reduces sodium but spares potassium, which is an improvement over other types of diuretic medications. Spironolactone is also indicated for the treatment of hair loss, helping to reduce androgen activity and slow hair loss through its anti-androgenic effects. Taken orally, it is sometimes prescribed for use in conjunction with topical minoxidil. However, in women with AGA, spironolactone does not promote the regrowth of hair. This drug works by blocking the androgen receptor and slowing the body's biological manufacturing process (biosynthesis) responsible for producing androgen hormone. It has been used effectively as a treatment for acne and hirsutism, and other types of alopecia in women, but scientists are not convinced of the drug's efficacy in correcting female pattern hair loss. One study of eighty women between the ages of 12 and 79 showed no significant differences in improvement between a control group that was not treated and women who received spironolactone. The overall results of this study were fifty=fifty, showing that 44 percent of women experienced hair growth and 44 percent experienced no improvement throughout the treatment period.

Spironolactone works as an anti-androgen agent by blocking the androgen receptor and reducing androgen production, as well as inhibiting the action of the enzyme that converts androgen in the hair follicle to its more aggressive cousin, DHT, which is directly involved in the hair loss associated with androgenetic alopecia. Side effects when taking spironolactone may include frequent urination even during the night, dizziness, and elevated potassium levels, which can affect the heart rate and other body functions. The elevated potassium occurs because the recommended dosage for treating hair loss is 200 mg per day, higher than that for treating hypertension, and high enough to increase potassium levels and produce side effects such as cramps and diarrhea. Women may also experience irregular periods while on this drug. Generally speaking, the lower the dosage, the fewer the side effects. However, because evidence of correcting hair loss is lacking with spironolactone, and unwanted side effects are known to develop, it may not be the first choice for treating hair loss in women, even though improvement has been seen in alopecia in several small studies investigating androgen excess in women.

DRUG THERAPIES FOR SCARRING ALOPECIA (CICATRICIAL ALOPECIA)

Cicatricial or scarring alopecia, which is characterized by follicle damage and permanent hair loss, requires aggressive treatment to prevent further damage and extensive losses. The type of treatment will vary based on what is causing the cicatricial alopecia and whether inflammation of the follicles is present, as in folliculitis, infections such as lichen planopilaris or pseudopelade, and dissecting cellulitis. Corticosteroids may be used in topical preparations or by injecting them into the inflamed areas. Antimalarial drugs are sometimes used for cicatricial alopecia. Malaria is caused by a parasite, but certain drugs that help kill the malarial parasite or prevent its growth are able to do the same with scarring alopecia that is caused by fungal or bacterial infection. The common antimalarial drugs (e.g., atovaquone, doxycycline, mefloquine and primaquine) have side effects such as nausea and dizziness but no serious side effects. They are not usually given to pregnant women. Another possible treatment is isotretinoin, a vitamin A fraction used effectively in treating acne; however, its use is limited because isotretinoin has been shown to cause birth defects and therefore it is not indicated for use in women of child-bearing age. If inflammation is shown to be caused by the presence of certain types of white cells (e.g., neutrophils or eosinophils), treatment may depend on the use of antibiotics. Autoimmune processes may be addressed by using a form of chemotherapy that suppresses overactivity of the immune system (immunosuppressants such as methotrexate). Because of the irreversible nature of cicatricial alopecia, diagnosing and treating it should be trusted to a physician who is highly experienced in treating this form of alopecia. Hair replacement procedures may be necessary for some individuals whose scarring of the scalp has produced irreversible balding. (See chapter 6.)

TOPICAL TREATMENTS AND DRUG THERAPIES FOR ALOPECIA AREATA

Corticosteroids are the principle treatment for alopecia areata in patients older than age ten and into adulthood, either applied topically to the affected areas of the scalp, injected as a solution into the bald spots (intralesional steroids), or taken orally for a systemic effect in the most severely affected patients. None of these corticosteroid treatments works consistently to achieve successful results in all patients, either to halt the condition or to encourage the regrowth of hair. Oral or systemic corticosteroids (e.g., methylprednisolone) have been associated with side effects such as reducing the quality of bone tissue, which reduces bone strength and integrity; side effects, relapse rate, and long treatment periods discourage use of systemic corticosteroids. Similarly, cyclosporine, an oral antibiotic, has been effective in treating alopecia areata, but possible side effects, a high recurrence rate, and long treatment have limited its use by prescribing physicians. In an unusual antagonistic approach, topical immunotherapy is delivered directly to the scalp by applying certain chemicals that are known allergens. When these are applied to the skin topically, they deliberately provoke an allergic reaction that has been shown to encourage hair growth. These drugs are called *contact sensitizers* and they are considered to be the most effective treatment available for the most severe and chronic cases of alopecia areata, reversing the condition in 40 to 60 percent of individuals. Another new category of oral medications called *biologics* are being tested (see page 113) for their ability to halt autoimmune processes and foster regrowth of hair in women who may have alopecia areata.

Anthralin Cream

Anthralin (0.5 to 1 percent) is a topical drug in cream form that is applied to the scalp for 20 minutes to start, then increasing the contact time weekly until a maximum of one hour. It is removed from the scalp with mineral oil, followed by washing with soap and water. It is only intended for scalp application, not for eyebrows. About 20 to 25 percent of patients can expect regrowth of hair with short-contact anthralin therapy. Some changes may be seen in immune system function, but the treatment has been proven to be safe and effective. Irritation, scaling, folliculitis, and swelling of lymph nodes may develop as side effects. The skin will likely be stained temporarily. The use of minoxidil topical solution in conjunction with anthralin applications is believed to be more effective than either topical drug used alone. In patients who respond favorably, new hair growth can be seen within three months.

Injectable Corticosteroids

Corticosteroid drugs are available in injectable solutions (intralesional triamcinolone acetonide) that can be delivered under the skin to balding areas of the scalp. Injections are considered to be first choice of therapy for adults with less than 50 percent of the scalp affected by alopecia areata. Injections are repeated every four to six weeks and regrowth is seen in four to eight weeks in the areas injected. Treatment is painful and larger volumes of the drug may cause thickening (atrophy) of scalp tissue. Not all patients respond and treatment is usually stopped if no regrowth occurs within six months after the first treatment. Injecting steroids does not change the status of the alopecia areata condition itself and hair can resume shedding even after regrowth has been seen.

Oral Glucocorticoids Combined with Minoxidil and Steroid Injections

Recommended only for patients with extensive or rapidly spreading alopecia areata, oral prednisone is typically given in 40 mg doses each day for the first week, reducing the dose by 5 mg each week until 20 mg is reached, and then adjusting dosage by 5 mg every three days until a 5 mg dose is given the last three days. This gradual tapering in dosage is standard for glucocorticoid therapy. Lesser amounts may be recommended for individuals with less extensive alopecia areata. Prednisone can be given in conjunction with the topical application of 5 percent minoxidil. Additionally, an injectable steroid drug (intralesional triamcinolone acetonide, described previously) can be delivered into the bald areas every four to six weeks. When alopecia areata is treated with these combined therapies, results are shown to be better than using any of the therapies alone.

Immunotherapy for the Scalp

The use of known allergens—contact sensitizing drugs that cause an allergic reaction—is a newer type of immunotherapy delivered directly to the scalp. These immunomodulating drugs have been shown to positively affect the immune system response that result from autoimmune alopecia areata and to produce regrowth of hair. Physicians and researchers have reported a success rate of 40 to 60 percent in patients who have 25 to 99 percent of the scalp affected. As such, this type of drug may become the most effective drug yet for treating chronic alopecia areata. Positive response to treatment of alopecia totalis and alopecia universalis has been shown to be as much as 25 percent.

Treatment involves applying solutions of the drugs diphencypron or squaric acid dibutyl ester directly to one side of the scalp at a time in small areas, continuing with weaker solutions applied once a week thereafter to the same side of the head. Two days after each treatment, the patient will remove the drug coating by washing the scalp. The doctor will observe the patient's response to each week's treatment to determine the appropriate strength for the next week's treatment. Patients will experience mild itching or irritation, redness (erythema), and scaling in response to the treatment, but these responses actually indicate a favorable response. Motivated patients will likely endure the minor discomforts.

MEDICAL TREATMENT FOR TELOGEN EFFLUVIUM

Removing the causative factor or treating an underlying disease or condition is the first line of treatment for telogen effluvium. In some situations, where the trigger for TE is known, removing the trigger and waiting for the hair growth cycle to correct itself is the best approach. After a trauma to the body like surgery, for example, some hair loss or shedding may be present, but as the body recovers from the trauma, normal hair growth will usually resume. Similarly, when a medication is known to trigger hair loss, changing the medication (e.g., antidepressants) may be all that is needed to restore the normal hair growth cycle. Hormone imbalances are known to affect the hair growth cycle and may trigger TE after childbirth and during menopause; correcting the hormone balance or waiting for the imbalance to correct on its own is usually all that's needed to stop shedding. In other forms of TE, however, the cause or trigger may not be obvious or may be difficult to identify. The dermatologist may then prescribe one of the same hair growth stimulating drugs used for androgenetic alopecia such as minoxidil, which has been shown to directly result in hair growth. This may produce hair growth while the underlying cause for TE is being sought through diagnostic testing. Once the underlying cause is identified and treatment begins, the physician may discontinue minoxidil.

Essentially, because so many different illnesses and triggers can lead to telogen effluvium, treatment depends on making an accurate diagnosis of the underlying condition or correctly identifying the trigger for TE so that appropriate treatment can be determined.

REVERSING DRUG-INDUCED OR RADIATION-INDUCED ANAGEN EFFLUVIUM

Because drug-induced or radiation-induced anagen effluvium is a temporary condition and not scarring, normal hair growth will be restored when the drug or radiation therapy is discontinued and no other treatment is needed. The normal anagen phase in the hair growth cycle can begin as early as two weeks after the termination of treatment and actual hair growth may be seen within a month. Because the hair follicles have remained intact, regrowth will be of normal density for the individual, but sometimes hair color may be different in the new growth.

Although no treatment other than terminating the chemotherapy or radiation is usually applied, shortening the period of hair loss caused by chemotherapy is a treatment goal for some individuals. Topical minoxidil is sometimes used on the scalp during chemotherapy or radiation treatments to reduce the duration of baldness even though it will not prevent it. In some cases, the period of baldness can be shortened by up to fifty days. Applying a pressure cuff around the scalp during the administration of chemotherapy will not prevent anagen arrest but will slow it down. Similarly, cold treatments (local hypothermia) are used in European countries and less widely in the United States to decrease the blood flow in the scalp by cooling it, which slows the delivery of medication to that part of the body. In a cold treatment, ice packs or a hood with ice-water inserts are applied to the scalp during the administration of chemotherapy drugs. This puts hair follicles into a state of suspension before they come into contact with the drug itself. Therefore, hair follicles do not take up the drug and are not damaged, effectively reducing anagen arrest and subsequent hair loss. Patients with leukemia, lymphoma, and other forms of blood cancer (hematologic malignancies) are usually not able to receive this type of cold treatment since the scalp is often a target for malignant cells circulating in the blood, and the drug would therefore not destroy malignant cells in the scalp's circulation as intended.

ANTIFUNGAL TREATMENT FOR TINEA CAPITIS—RINGWORM OF THE SCALP

Tinea capitis is a very persistent, highly contagious fungal infection of the scalp that is usually treated with oral antifungal medications such as griseofulvin, itraconazole, terbinafine, or fluconazole. As new drugs are introduced, side effects appear to be reduced further. The doctor will be able to recommend the appropriate antifungal for each patient. Although antifungals can be effective, treatment can be long term because of the tenacity of fungi and likely recurrence of the fungus. In some cases of kerion, the most severe type of tinea capitis infection with greater hair loss, oral steroid drugs may be recommended to reduce inflammation and prevent significant scarring. Home remedies decidedly don't work to stop the fungus from spreading. To reduce or prevent spreading, the affected area must be kept clean using a medicated shampoo that contains selenium sulfide, or other antifungal ingredient. Otherwise, the affected area should be kept cool and dry. All personal items such as clothing, headgear, combs, and brushes should be kept separate to protect other members of the household. Family members and household pets should be examined and treated if any signs of fungus infection are seen.

NATURAL HERBAL OR NEUTRACEUTICAL TREATMENTS FOR HAIR LOSS

Herbal or neutraceutical treatments for encouraging hair growth are preferred and sought by some individuals rather than to use pharmaceutical drug therapies or surgical procedures to correct their hair loss problems. The reason given most often is simply a preference to use naturally occurring biochemicals found in plant sources rather than synthetic chemical formulations. Most herbal or neutraceutical hair loss treatments, similar to the conventional medical treatments described earlier, are intended to prevent the formation of dihydrotestosterone (DHT), the form of testosterone found in the scalp of men and women who have noticeable hair loss of the androgenetic alopecia or pattern baldness type. Many herbal formulas have been developed to inhibit DHT formation and most of them contain one or more of the same components: biotin, saw palmetto, gotu kola, and muira puama. Some of these constituents and their nutritive properties include the following (Balch, 2002):

Biotin—Part of the B complex of vitamins, it is important in the utilization of other B vitamins and in cell growth and fatty acid production; essential to metabolism of fats, proteins, and carbohydrates; and necessary for healthy hair and skin (100 milligrams daily may prevent hair loss in some individuals). Deficiency of biotin can contribute to anemia, depression, hair loss, inflammation, insomnia, muscular pain, and loss of appetite.

Vitamin B⁶ (pyridoxine)—Helps maintain sodium/potassium balance, necessary for production of hydrochloric acid and absorption of fats and proteins, promotes red blood cell formation, and essential to nervous system functioning and normal brain function and for the synthesis of RNA and DNA. Vitamin B⁶ also is vital to heart health by aiding in the prevention of atherosclerosis and inhibiting the formation of homocysteine, which attacks heart muscle. Deficiency of B⁶ can result in acne, arthritis, depression, headaches, poor wound healing, inflammation, flaky skin, hair loss, weak memory, and hearing problems.

Zinc—An essential mineral important to prostate function, growth of reproductive organs, immune system functioning, antioxidant activity, wound healing, protein synthesis, and bone and collagen formation. A zinc deficiency can cause or contribute to acne, delayed sexual maturation, impotence, infertility, fatigue, hair loss, thinning of nails, prostate problems, and slow wound healing.

Saw palmetto—Contains capric, caproic, lauric, oleic, and palmitic acids. It stimulates appetite, enhances sexual function, and inhibits the production of dihydrotestosterone—a hormone that contributes to enlarging the prostate gland and is a factor in pattern hair loss.

Gotu kola—Contains catechol, epicatechol, magnesium, theobromine, and vitamin K. It aids in eliminating excess fluids, decreases fatigue, helps balance hormones and enhance sexual function, stimulates central nervous system, and aids heart and liver function and blood circulation.

Rosemary—Contains bitters, camphor, carnosic acid, cineole, essential oils, pinene, resin, and tannins. It stimulates circulation and digestion, relaxes digestive organs, helps prevent liver toxicity, has antitumor properties, aids in treating headaches, helps normalize blood pressure, and acts as an antibacterial agent, astringent, and decongestant.

Another common botanical ingredient of herbal formulas, called muira puama (liriosma ovata), comes from the Amazon region and has stirred up controversy elsewhere. It purportedly contains alkaloids, esters, plant sterols, fatty acids, and phytosterols. It is reported widely on the Internet that muira puama is "in use worldwide" to enhance hormone balance in both sexes and to improve sexual function, boost energy levels and general health, and improve nervous system functioning. No information is shown about the value of this botanical in hair loss formulas. It is known as the "Viagra of the Amazon" and it is not approved by the FDA as a product or an ingredient for any indication; neither are published studies available in support of this botanical constituent's use.

Other ingredients of herbal formulas may include magnesium, zinc, nettle, uva-ursi, chamomile, and eleuthero (Siberian ginseng). Some herbal manufacturers provide shampoos and conditioners to treat the scalp topically while the individual also takes an oral herbal formula. Some preparations even include minoxidil. One herbal formula gaining some attention—not all good attention—is Provillus, whose manufacturer claims has been shown to be safe and effective in use as well as cost effective. The only ingredient in Provillus that has been proven to be safe and effective for use in men to treat male pattern baldness is minoxidil. Although many testimonials supporting Provillus can be found on the Internet, the American Hair Loss Association (AHLA), in its professional blog (http://blog.americanhairloss.org/category/provillus/), says, "Provillus is nothing more than an overpriced dietary supplement along with repackaged generic minoxidil and azelaic acid."

To be fair to Provillus, let's see what's in it. The blend of herbs, minerals, and vitamins reported to be in Provillus includes saw palmetto, gotu kola, nettles, magnesium, zinc sulfate, Siberian ginseng, vitamin B^6, pumpkin seed, and muira puama root. You can see some of these ingredients in the constituent list above. While herbalists can provide a rationale for the biochemical action of most of these constituents, the American Hair Loss Association blog states that none of these nutritional supplements is approved by the FDA for any medical purpose let alone prevention or treatment of hair loss. I present both positions so that you can be aware of opinions and options. Herbal and nutritional sources of healing have been trusted for centuries in cultures not our own. Enlightened holistic practitioners around the world recommend them and it's easy to find testimonials from satisfied users. I'm happy to say that I have trusted herbal anti-inflammatory tinctures for nearly fifteen years to effectively treat joint pain from rheumatoid arthritis and to protect liver function while taking an FDA-approved drug that is known to damage liver tissue. However, other than using a rosemary shampoo and conditioner to make my hair appear fuller, I haven't used herbal formulas for hair loss, so I can give no personal opinion here.

The AHLA blog reminds us that regardless of the claims and accolades by users, there are only two products proven to stop the progression of hair loss and to regrow hair: minoxidil and finasteride. However, the association adds that "if a product is not approved by the FDA or does not carry the AHLA certification seal, don't waste your time or money on it." This sounds like a strong position; after all, it's a blog—a chance to sound off. However, this opinion does not mean that taking essential nutrients will not help create healthy follicles or that herbs will not help balance hormones, which in theory could be adjunctive therapy while FDA-approved minoxidil does its work. What it does mean is that you have to know your sources of information. If the blog you consult is called "Balding Tony," you're getting an opinion only; if it's a blog posted by the American Hair Loss Association, one would expect to be getting objective information from professionals. You will have to decide for yourself who—and which products and manufacturers—you are prepared to trust.

More information about herbal and nutritional topical treatments can be found in chapter 7.

A RANGE OF DRUGS IN THE PHARMACEUTICAL PIPELINE

Toward the end of the last century, only a handful of researchers were studying hair biology and hair diseases. In the early part of the twenty-first century, we know that five times as many researchers are looking into the various forms of alopecia, including the hereditary form called androgenetic alopecia. New technologies such as genomics and proteomics are available for studying genetics and gene mutations, for example, which may help to better understand the mechanisms involved in hair loss and to target specific drug therapies to treat them. People with rare alopecias may also benefit from the time being spent investigating hair biology and potential biologic treatments, even though significantly more research is devoted to such life-threatening diseases as diabetes, heart disease, and cancer.

Experimental drugs to block drug-induced hair loss are in the process of being developed; however, the major concern is that any drug used to prevent drug-induced hair loss may simultaneously protect malignant cells in the skin, allowing them to spread.

Non-FDA-approved drugs for hair loss include cyproterone acetate (available in Europe but not in the United States), progesterone, cimetidine (Tagamet), and other nonprescription and herbal products.

This does not mean that they do not contribute to hair growth, but that sufficient safety and efficacy has not been demonstrated to encourage hair growth after losses occur.

Biologics are a new group of drugs being investigated in clinical trials, especially for the treatment of autoimmune disease and autoimmune processes that can result in certain diseases or hair loss conditions such as autoimmune alopecia (alopecia areata). The principle behind biologics is similar to "hair of the dog," which is that receiving a tiny bit more of a substance that causes illness may be enough to stop the process underlying the illness. Biologics are tiny bits of protein that have been shown to interrupt the activity of immune system cells. The pharmaceutical strategy is that injection of biologics into the system of an individual with autoimmune disease will retard the immune system activity. In the case of autoimmune alopecia, this means possible regrowth of hair. Dermatologists are eager to know the results of these clinical trials because they could make a significant difference in outcomes for alopecia patients.

STRESS REDUCTION AS A TREATMENT FOR HAIR LOSS

You undoubtedly remember reading that stress was a factor in nearly all of the nonscarring forms of alopecia. Although not a cause in every form of alopecia, it's able to aggravate the hair loss condition in most cases. And who among us wouldn't be aggravated by the very thought of hair loss—the psychological effects of losing hair, or even thinning hair, can have a significant emotional impact. Part of this may be a result of the perception that so few women lose hair compared to men and that hair loss in women is not at all acceptable, whereas it's normal in men and totally accepted socially. This is, of course, not entirely true, if we look at the numbers of women affected, but perception is sometimes the reality.

A group of researchers led by Dr. Ina Hadshiew in 2004 compiled a list of negative effects described by hair loss patients seeking identification and treatment of their conditions. The list is a review of patient-perceived effects published in the work of other dermatology researchers studying hair loss patients. Among the list of feelings experienced and self-reported by patients are these, listed alphabetically with no distinction in the frequency of feelings:

- Anger
- Depression
- Discomfort
- Disgrace
- Disgust
- Dissatisfaction with body image
- Embarrassment
- Feeling of being older
- Fright
- Frustration
- Helplessness
- Humiliation
- Loss of self-confidence
- Powerlessness
- Reduced social acceptance
- Reduced worth
- Sadness
- Self-consciousness
- Self-hate
- Sense of inadequacy
- Shame
- Social stress
- Unhappy about appearance
- Worry

Faced with any of these emotions, women with hair loss sometimes begin to limit their social activities, significantly affecting their quality of life and sometimes their work and activities of daily life. Some women go into hiding altogether, whereas others hide just until they find a suitable wig or begin treatment of some kind. Women who develop drug-induced alopecia as a result of receiving chemotherapy or taking certain other therapeutic drugs are often devastated by the accompanying hair loss—sometimes facing complete baldness until their course of treatment is over. And it doesn't always help to know that hair growth will resume after drug therapy. Some women even refuse potentially life-saving chemotherapy treatment because they cannot accept even temporary baldness. Ripe with a range of upsetting emotional reactions, many people with hair loss seek the support of a therapist or a support group for people with all types of alopecia. And newer strategies for treating any type of alopecia include addressing both clinical and psychological symptoms of hair loss. Support groups and professional counseling are becoming easier to find, with national hair loss associations leading the way with appropriate resources. More information is available on the National Alopecia Areata Foundation Web site (www.naaf.org).

Another reason that prescribing physicians and national alopecia organizations are supporting the use of stress reduction resources is that clinical studies of men and women with hair loss have shown that medical treatments produce more effective results when psychological treatment is applied simultaneously. Medically, acute or chronic stress can be a causative factor in types of hair loss that originally stem from an endocrine, metabolic, or immunological cause, implicating especially the hormonally triggered androgenetic alopecia and the autoimmune androgenetic alopecia. And we also know that traumatic events can produce the type of hair loss called telogen effluvium and that this hair loss typically reverses when time has passed and the stressful effects of the trauma have been treated. Hair restoration physicians also believe that stress aggravates various types of alopecia, especially the most common female AGA and chronic telogen effluvium (CTE) that manifest in middle-aged women, so it seems to make absolute sense to include stress reduction as part of overall treatment. If stress is known to cause or to aggravate alopecia, imagine the full impact of causative stress combined with the stress associated with losing hair—that is, the presence of any of the patient-perceived feelings reported above.

Stress reduction techniques include deep breathing or yogic breathing; the practice of yoga, tai chi, or qigong; progressive muscle relaxation; creative visualization; meditation; or programs that teach the relaxation response. Exercise itself is known to contribute to managing stress. Health and wellness centers around the country are offering various types of programs that are designed to help people learn new ways to process what happens during ordinary life and how to handle the ups and downs in a more balanced and comfortable way. Our world is fast paced and stressors abound at work, at home, and in our personal and business relationships. Some of us are more prone to stressors than others and learning how to ride the waves of our lives can be of great benefit to our overall health—and to the influence of stress on specific health problems such as hair loss.

So, while we're trying to manage hair loss, we may also need the benefits of managing stress—taking charge of our own emotions, thoughts, and how we choose to address our problems. Start investigating the type of stress management that may work for you by: (1) finding a therapist or counselor near you; (2) seeking a class on yoga, tai chi, qigong, or meditation; (3) checking out your local health care institutions (hospitals, clinics, or public health organizations) to see if they have a stress reduction program; or (4) asking your doctor to refer you to a program in your area known to help manage stress. Your doctor may also be able to recommend ways to deal with the effects that stress might be having on your health and your hair loss. Stress takes a toll on your body in ways you can't always see, such as by reducing your immune system functioning and leaving you more vulnerable to illness. But you can see the effects on your hair. Since stress has been shown to be an important factor in hair loss, regardless of what type of alopecia you may have, managing your stress can surely contribute to managing your hair loss. You can take charge of that starting right now.

CHAPTER 6

SURGICAL HAIR RESTORATION AND LASER TECHNIQUES

Hair transplantation, identifying a good candidate; scalp reduction and scalp flap surgery; hair growth enhancement with low-level laser therapy; the future of hair replacement (hair cloning, hair multiplication, genetic engineering and other management options)

SURGICAL AND LASER TECHNIQUES TO RESTORE LOST HAIR

Restoring lost hair involves making personal choices. Will you take medications or undergo surgery? Do you want the hairstyle you've always had, or something new? Are you willing to camouflage your hair loss rather than replace it? There are many questions and, as you will see, many different types of solutions.

In this chapter you'll find descriptions of some of the leading hair replacement and hair growth enhancement procedures performed by qualified medical practitioners in independent surgical centers or hospital-based hair restoration surgery centers. The idea is to gather enough information about hair replacement options to help you make a choice between medications or replacement, between surgical or laser techniques, between newer transplant procedures or older scalp reduction surgeries, and finally, between restoring your own hair or relying on cosmetic solutions. The variables on which the decision depends include the cause and extent of your hair loss, your suitability as a transplant candidate, the condition of your scalp and follicles, the density of your hair at the time of surgery, and, most of all, your preferences and objectives. Do you want to have thicker hair? Do you want to replace lost hair or fill in balding spots? Do you want a one-time, fix-all procedure? These are only some of the questions you might want to consider. Your doctor or your dermatologist or transplant surgeon will help you with the answers and can be of great support during the decision-making phase as well as ongoing support during the treatment you finally select.

SURGICAL PROCEDURES FOR REPLACING LOST HAIR

Not all women who are losing hair because of androgenetic alopecia want to try medications as a way to increase the anagen phase of the growth cycle—it seems like the long route. Although drug therapies may work for some, hair growth remedies have recognized drawbacks as well. To review, minoxidil is the only medication currently available for stimulation of hair growth in women (finasteride is approved for use in men only). And minoxidil, as we've learned, must be used forever or the thinning returns. Spironolactone has helped many women, particularly women whose hair loss started years before menopause, but many months can pass before any results are seen, and the final results are not dramatic. As a double whammy against progressive hair loss, hormone replacement medications are sometimes recommended *with* spironolactone for postmenopausal women—and sometimes the combination works well, depending on how much thinning has occurred. And, topping off the drawbacks, only one third of all people—men and women—using hair growth stimulants actually see satisfying results. Rather than be disappointed, or having to commit to using a topical solution or oral drug therapy for the rest of their lives, some women opt for hair replacement surgery.

By all reports from medical and consumer sources, modern surgical hair replacement procedures have been producing good to excellent results for qualified candidates and are constantly being improved to create the most natural hair replacement results possible. Yes, the procedures can involve time, patience, and a limited amount of pain, as well as significant dollars, but satisfactory results are realized more quickly than they are with medications, and the results are permanent, ruling out lifetime treatment as the only option.

We have to remember, though, that surgical procedures don't guarantee against losing more hair as people age, and surgeons performing these procedures sometimes recommend using minoxidil as part of long-term follow-up. Managing the balding of androgenetic alopecia, for example, which can involve an unpredictable progression of hair loss, means monitoring changes in the individual's hair pattern that might include a decreasing amount of permanent hair as the individual gets older. For some individuals, this could mean thinning hair and, for others, new balding areas. In either case, the hair restoration specialist will undoubtedly counsel patients and help them address these issues as they develop. It's important to go into surgery

118

with realistic expectations about what the surgery will correct and what can happen in the long term.

Making the decision to undergo surgery is an individual matter. It's important for each person to seek a qualified physician hair restoration specialist, be fully evaluated as a candidate for surgical hair replacement, and get a good understanding of the recommended surgery before going into the process so that expectations are realistic. Because medications to restore hair growth have had only limited success in women in the first place, and require a lifetime commitment in the second place, a onetime hair replacement procedure seems to be the more attractive alternative cosmetically and psychologically. Modern hair transplant procedures have been refined significantly in the last twenty years and are reported to be the best option for people who have a good crop of healthy donor hair. Although hair grafting is considered to be the established method of choice for hair restoration, older surgical procedures such as scalp reduction are still being performed. Either method can provide good permanent results for people who do not want to rely on medications alone.

ARE YOU A GOOD CANDIDATE FOR HAIR TRANSPLANTATION?

Once your physician has confirmed that your hair loss condition is female AGA, hair transplantation is a treatment option. Always remember that it's your option, not the physician's; you're the only one who chooses how you wish to treat your hair loss after you've reviewed all the medical, surgical, and cosmetic options available to you and have discussed your hair loss condition fully with your doctor. If you decide on surgery, you'll want to consider the details of the procedure and the recovery period, the cost of the treatment, time involved, and any potential complications or side effects. Most important, perhaps, you'll consider the outcome: how your hair will look after your surgery.

The ideal candidate for transplantation has: (1) confirmed female AGA, (2) a hair loss pattern that can be treated by transplantation, (3) healthy follicles, (4) enough donor hair of sufficient quality to make a transplant effective, and (5) has expectations that can be satisfied with transplantation. The physician hair replacement specialist will also consider cosmetic factors such as hair color and texture, whether your hair is straight or curly, and the contrast between your skin color and hair color. Any of these factors could affect the final result of transplantation. If you are being considered for hair transplantation, you will also have a full evaluation by the hair replacement specialist or surgeon.

EVALUATION BEFORE TRANSPLANTATION

The process of hair restoration by surgical transplant begins as any other surgical transplant procedure would—with an evaluation of the hair loss problem and the potential donor solution. The back and sides of the head will be examined for potentially good harvesting sites where hair is thick and healthy and follicles are in good condition. Hair follicles at the back and sides of the head are androgen independent, meaning that they are known not to shed as a result of genetic programming, and therefore these sites usually have the best hair density for successful harvesting of donor follicles. Even after these follicles are transplanted, they retain their androgen independent, nonshedding characteristic, which precludes hair loss and helps maintain hair density for the patient's lifetime—providing both a permanent solution to the hair loss problem and a natural solution that complements the patient's own hair.

Hair transplantation procedures are typically performed in hair restoration centers under local anesthesia delivered to the scalp. The procedures can be extremely long, ranging from several hours to an entire working day, depending on how many follicles are being transplanted. Nevertheless, highly motivated patients are not discouraged by this, knowing that they will remain fairly comfortable, and can watch television during the procedure or even take naps—and, above all, being confident that the result will be worth their time and patience.

HAIR TRANSPLANT PROCEDURES

Hair transplants are not new; the first report of a successful transplant procedure was published in 1952. Transplants of the type described in that report were performed over the next thirty years to achieve permanent restoration of hair in people of all ages who had lost hair from various causes. However, there is a world of difference between today's procedures and those of the 1950s—not only in the technique itself, but in the results. Older transplant procedures used a method called the *plug technique*, which called for large grafts of hair to be removed by round punches about the size of a pencil eraser. The final result, besides being associated with a bleeding scalp and pain, unfortunately looked "plugged in." Even though hair was now growing in spots that had previously been bald, telltale signs of surgery were visible on the scalp, giving the hair itself the appearance of unnatural "doll's hair" protruding from holes.

In the transplantation techniques used today, whole follicular units are extracted and transplanted. Newer micro-graft procedures differ from the older punch procedures by using large numbers, often thousands, of very small grafts (mini-micro grafts), so tiny that they heal on their own with no bleeding at all, and with only mild discomfort that can be easily treated with medications when needed. It's a whole different head game. Patients are able to resume normal activities twenty-four hours after transplant surgery, and can even shower and shampoo their hair within a day or two.

The modern procedures that were introduced in the mid-1990s are called follicular unit transplantation (FUT) and follicular unit extraction (FUE). In FUT, donor hairs are obtained from the lower back of the individual's scalp where androgen-independent hairs can be found that don't shed. The procedure is performed by hair transplant surgeons skilled in removing the donor hairs and also, more and more these days, creative surgeons who have some sense of the aesthetics of hair replacement. Depending on where the losses have occurred, the frontal hairline may need replacement as well as the top and sides. If the surgeon is without a sense of hair aesthetics, the individual could potentially wind up with a permanent bad hair day. This is not likely to happen, though, since hair transplant surgeons are constantly improving their techniques, both in the harvesting of hairs and the implanting procedure, as well as in creating a visually pleasing hairline.

Hair transplant procedures are performed while the patient sits in a chair not unlike the standard dentist's chair or the familiar recliner. The entire scalp will first be cleaned with antiseptic solutions and both the donor and recipient areas will then be anesthetized by injecting a numbing solution (usually a combination of lidocaine and epinephrine) under the skin. Another drug called triamcinolone may also be injected into the recipient site to help reduce postoperative swelling and to prevent any temporary loss of hair (telogen effluvium) that could occur because of surgical trauma to the scalp. A mild oral sedative or a gas such as nitrous oxide may be given to reduce the discomfort that may be caused by the administration of anesthesia to the scalp.

The first step of the follicular unit transplant procedure is to remove, or harvest, a thin strip of hair from the back or sides of the scalp, immediately stitching the harvested area to close it. The donor area will not show after the strip is removed because it is covered over by the length of hair growing immediately above it. The strip of hair includes the follicles from which each hair grows. These are examined under a microscope (dissecting microscope), allowing the surgeon to extract several follicular units at a time with their inclusive hairs, which are reserved for grafting. After this meticulous procedure of selecting and harvesting individual follicular units, the units are placed in a special holding solution to preserve the integrity of the tissue, and then are stored under refrigeration until the surgeon is ready to place them in the balding or thinning areas of the patient's head.

Miniscule incisions, or graft incision sites, are then made in the patient's scalp where coverage is needed. These tiny recipient sites are made by using a thin blade or very small needle. The pattern or distribution of incisions, along with the depth and angles of the incisions, has a lot to do with the final result. The goal is to create new hair growth that is as natural as the patient's own hair growth. This typically involves making larger incisions farther back on the scalp for greater density of final growth, and smaller incisions for single hairs in the frontal areas of the scalp where the hair needs to gradually increase in density from thin to thicker in a sort of "feathered" effect. The surgeon is almost required to be an artist in the design and placement of the new follicular units, understanding that the pattern, depth, and angle will make a difference in the appearance of the replacement hair growth. Surgeons often mark out a grid on the patient's scalp to help ensure even distribution of grafts and appropriate density for each area being grafted.

Follicular units are inserted, or grafted, individually into the scalp in the prepared recipient sites, matching the differently sized follicle units with up to four hairs in each to the different recipient sites and creating a tight fit for each unit. Grafting is a meticulous placement process requiring great skill of the surgeon so that hair follicle injury is avoided and that the proper angle is achieved with each graft placed. The better each follicular unit fits, the faster the site will heal and the sooner hair growth will start. The frontal hairline (anterior hairline) is not usually affected on women, but if the frontal area is thinner and requires some transplantation, special attention is required. Transplanted follicles must create an aesthetically pleasing and natural hairline, not one that starts abruptly or unnaturally on the forehead. As described, this will mean using fine, single-hair follicular-unit grafts to create a slightly feathered area leading into the more dense hair on the sides and top of the head. A skilled surgeon, with artistic sensibilities, can produce a natural head of hair and a very happy postoperative result for the patient.

The follicular unit extraction (FUE) procedure is similar to FUT except for the way the donor follicles are harvested. In FUE, the donor follicles are obtained by first shaving the back of the head and then removing individual follicular units with a small circular incision. The donor follicular units are removed from the scalp one at a time, leaving such tiny incisions that they easily close by themselves within a week after surgery. The donor follicles are transplanted the same way as in the FUT procedure described earlier. The procedure has proven to be a useful alternative to FUT if, for some reason, harvesting follicles in a strip is not an option for a particular patient.

After either the FUT or FUE procedure has been performed, the scalp and all recipient sites are cleaned off with either a saline or hydrogen peroxide solution. Antibiotic cream or ointment will be applied but dressings are not needed. The transplants will be visible on the scalp for a week or so. Postoperative care may include oral antibiotics and light spraying of the scalp with a hydrogen peroxide solution. Medication is given as needed for any pain or discomfort experienced while the incision sites are healing. Except for avoiding strenuous exercise, transplant recipients can resume their normal daily activities—with or without a hat—and can expect to see hair growth in two to three months.

Complications are rare, and fortunately, so are poor results. Sometimes, if a physician has been urged by a patient to place a hairline too low, it can produce less than ideal aesthetic results; surgeons usually advise against this, but negotiation may result in a greater attempt to satisfy the patient's concerns and fill in a frontal area with grafts. In this case, a scalp reduction technique may be combined with transplantation to address concerns about frontal area hair loss. Telogen effluvium, temporary loss of existing hair due to the surgical trauma, is a possibility in some patients and all patients should be aware of this before going into the procedure (see "Telogen Effluvium," chapter 3). Most patients, however, will be enjoying a full head of hair in ten months or so, knowing that it is for the rest of their lives. It's easy to understand why hair transplantation is currently considered the gold standard of hair replacement methods. According to all reports, and regardless of favorable medical opinions, hair transplant recipients certainly seem satisfied and happy with their outcome.

Laser-Assisted Hair Transplantation

For a few years during the 1990s, laser hair transplants provided another surgical option. Surgeons tried using a laser beam to make the holes for grafting follicles, and although laser worked well enough as a cutting tool, hair growth results were mixed. Some surgeries resulted in scalp damage and scarring, and hair growth was not as good as hoped for after surgery. As a result, the procedure lost favor and laser-assisted transplants of this type are not performed any longer by physicians at major hair restoration centers.

Combination Treatments

If a patient has a significant area of hair loss but lacks sufficient donor hair for transplant, the restoration specialist may recommend combining limited hair transplantation with a certain type of hairstyling. Compromises can often be reached to satisfy both the medical/surgical requirements and the patient's expectations.

Other possible combinations include the use of minoxidil after transplantation to help address continuing hair loss in areas that were not transplanted, and scalp reduction or scalp flaps (see below) to address frontal hair loss when a pleasing aesthetic cannot be achieved for the frontal hairline with transplantation.

Combination treatments will always be negotiated between the physician and the patient until the best overall treatment option has been agreed on and the expected outcomes are understood.

Synthetic Hair Transplantation

Because of side effects reported in the 1970s, transplantation of synthetic hair is currently banned in the United States even though it has been done in other parts of the world for over thirty years. The recipients of synthetic hair are typically people who do not have sufficient donor hair for FUT and FUE procedures. Companies in Japan and Italy are manufacturing synthetic hair using polymer fibers. The use of these fibers is being investigated in ongoing clinical studies, so it is possible that we will see more widespread use of these fibers in the future.

Scalp Reduction and Scalp Flaps

At one time scalp reduction was performed widely to minimize areas of balding. Today, however, these surgical alternatives to hair transplants are still performed but are no match for follicular unit transplantation, which has enjoyed increased consumer demand as patient testimonials published on the Internet have increased interest in the procedure. The procedures known medically as scalp reduction and scalp flaps are usually performed for people who may not have enough healthy donor hair to allow them to be appropriate candidates for transplantation. They may also be performed when excessive scarring of the scalp has occurred or when a specific hair pattern must be restored. Scalp reduction and flaps are generally more aggressive types of surgery that carry a risk of scarring and can result in less-natural hair growth.

The principle behind scalp reduction is for the surgeon to gradually close up balding areas by cutting (excising) parts of the bald scalp and pulling together the surrounding scalp tissue to create sufficient hair coverage. By following various shapes of scalp excisions (ellipse, Y, crescent, and horseshoe shapes), according to the elasticity of the patient's scalp, different patterns of hair loss can be minimized or eliminated entirely. Sometimes several surgeries are needed until the hair margins meet and the bare areas are filled. Techniques have definitely improved since the pretransplant days of the early 1980s to 1990. Scalp reduction can fairly quickly restore the individual's own head of hair—often a satisfying result even though scalp tissue may be temporarily thinned as a result.

To support a more effective result with scalp reduction techniques, sometimes the scalp area will be expanded prior to the reduction procedure. An expander or extender is placed into the scalp about six weeks prior to the surgery and regular injections of saline are used to progressively increase the scalp surface area.

In women, a high hairline and/or a prominent forehead or receding frontal hairline can be corrected by using a frontal hairline advancement procedure, often performed in conjunction with the brow lift procedure. It is performed in a way that avoids a noticeable scar and the patient enjoys the benefits of both a brow lift and an improved hairline through frontal scalp reduction.

Reduction procedures may have several complications such as misdirected hair—that is, hair growing in a direction that doesn't appear natural. Misdirected hair is usually the result of repetitive scalp reductions and the pulling together of mismatched areas of hair growth, with hairs growing at different angles. Other complications can include reduction in scalp hair density, an elevation in the frontal hairline, noticeable scarring of the scalp, and sometimes a "slot" defect at the back of the head where hair has parted unnaturally.

This slot defect is essentially an elongated scar that occurs when an area of scalp has been surgically removed and then has been closed with sutures. Scalp reductions are performed when the goal is to *reduce* the effects of alopecia rather than to eliminate them. Even with the possibility of complications, reduction usually provides good coverage in these cases. Scalp reductions are sometimes performed on certain balding patients in conjunction with grafting, especially if there is significant frontal hair loss, although this does not occur that often in women. A carefully designed and executed combination of grafting and scalp reduction can usually manage to correct both thinning and balding regardless of the pattern of loss.

Scalp Flaps for Frontal Hairline Replacement

Skin flaps, called *pedicle flaps* or TPO flaps (temporoparietal-occipital pedicle flaps), involve a series of exacting surgeries performed in stages to create complete, and almost instant, frontal hairlines in patients who are bald at the front of the scalp. Because female AGA does not usually affect the frontal hairline, women are less likely to have this procedure. However, it is included for discussion here to address a full range of treatments and the rare possibility that an individual reader will need frontal hairline restoration. Scalp flaps take existing hair growth from the hair fringe that curves around the bottom of the back of the head, the same region from which follicles are extracted in a strip for grafting. The patient must have excellent hair density and a supple scalp in the donor region to perform this unique surgical procedure. The surgery is particularly difficult and demanding for both the surgeon and the patient, and requires three separate procedures before it is complete. Excision of the flap and creation of adequate blood circulation (revascularization) is the first step; removing the flap and stapling the site closed is the second procedure performed a week later; and the third step, a week later still, is to transfer the flap to its new position at the front of the head and suture it onto the underlying scalp. Scarring can occur at the donor site on the back of the head; in women, hair growth above it may help to conceal the scar. Misdirected hair is as much of a problem with flaps as it is with scalp reduction, and additional ongoing hair loss can create an unnatural appearance around the flap itself. Because the procedure is complicated and its results aren't in keeping with techniques like follicular unit hair transplants that provide less noticeable hair replacement, pedicle flaps are seldom recommended or performed except in patients who are highly motivated to do it to replace significant frontal hair loss.

Complications with scalp flap procedures include swelling and bruising of the surgical site, significant scarring, and sometimes infection and stiffening (necrosis) of the ends of the flap because of poor blood circulation in the transplanted flap. With the latter condition, antibiotics are given orally and surgical repair of the flap may be needed. Cosmetically, the appearance of the frontal hair can be negatively affected by additional ongoing hair loss around the flap. Styling techniques or hairpieces can often help correct this problem.

LASER TECHNIQUES FOR HAIR GROWTH ENHANCEMENT

Photo-biotherapy is the science behind laser therapy. It refers to the absorption of laser light by tissue cells, resulting in enhanced cell metabolism and protein synthesis. The function and benefits of directed laser light have been demonstrated by clinical studies that showed several outstanding effects of laser treatment, such as increased anti-inflammatory effects, improved blood circulation to the skin, increased flow of lymph fluid in the body's lymphatic system, and decreased swelling. When promoting hair growth, the photo-biotherapy principle is applied by using low-level laser light to stimulate follicles on the scalp. Follicular cells are thereby encouraged to increase energy production and to reverse miniaturization. Not only does this process regenerate hair growth but thicker hair shafts are produced, which increases the appearance of fullness of the new hair growth. Laser treatments have been shown to achieve better results with thinning hair than they do in treating bald spots, and sometimes laser and hair growth medications like minoxidil are used together to maintain an adequate growth of new hair.

Low-Level Laser Therapy

Low-level laser therapy (LLLT) is a treatment method that uses a light source capable of generating light of a single wave-length. LLLT acts without creating thermal or photochemical activity in the cells or tissue being treated, and no heat, sound, or vibration is generated by devices that produce low-level laser beams. LLLT technology has been used to treat various disorders in which healing of tissue is needed, including wound healing (such as surgical wounds, open sores, and especially pressure sores or bedsores), burns, psoriasis, carpal tunnel syndrome, osteoarthritis, sprains, and lower back pain. Physicians, surgeons, practitioners of integrative medicine, naturopaths, physical therapists, licensed massage therapists, chiropractors, and athletic trainers, among others, have all used LLLT to heal injured or inflamed tissue.

Amazingly, the same laser light that helps to heal cells in body tissue can be employed to help grow hair. There is a logical scientific basis for this result if we remember the photo-biotherapy principle in which the basic function of tissue can be improved by the application of low-level laser. Scalp tissue can therefore benefit from LLLT, resulting in the stimulation of follicles to grow hair.

Laser technology has also been shown to be a *safe* treatment method, and for good reason. A laser diode generates laser light in the visible red light spectrum—or "red beam laser"—providing laser energy way below that of laser beams that are used to burn or cut tissue, as in the laser-assisted transplant surgery described previously. Low-level laser energy is also absorbed very slowly by human tissue. Knowing these things, surgeons specializing in hair replacement reasoned that laser technology might prove useful and safe in the treatment of hair loss. In the early 1990s, after experimenting with the technique, researchers published promising results of studies that employed laser treatments to regrow hair in volunteer subjects. Several types of large low-level laser units were in use at that time in European countries. After ten years of ongoing professional laser treatment for hair growth with these larger units, manufacturers in Europe and the United States developed and sought approval for handheld low-level laser devices. In 2007, the FDA gave a green light to marketing low-level laser devices, on the basis of safety alone, for treating androgenetic hair loss. Handheld low-level laser devices are classified by the FDA as a cosmetic product and companies introducing these products have not been permitted to make specific medical claims about the technique's effectiveness in regrowing hair. Patients, on the other hand, have been satisfied with the regrowth they've experienced and have talked about it freely in hair blogs and on Web sites. Although hair growth results vary from person to person, most patients report that satisfactory regrowth continues as long as they continue doing the laser treatments. If they stop the treatments, the growth eventually stops, indicating clearly that it's not permanent growth and that it's primarily the *appearance* of the hair that changes. Thin or miniaturized hair essentially becomes thicker and creates the appearance of a fuller head of hair. As far as the frequency of laser treatments that are needed, certain types of professional laser treatments produce longer-lasting results because of their more effective penetration of the scalp. However, people who elect to use the at-home LLLT products should understand from the beginning that their laser scalp treatment must become almost as regular as brushing and flossing their teeth—not daily necessarily, but surely a couple of treatments a week—if they want continued growth. Happily, with the availability of the new handheld laser "combs," regular at-home use is easy enough to accomplish.

Professional and Handheld At-Home Laser Units

The Revage Laser System is a large professional unit that features rotational phototherapy (RPT), referring to the underlying photo-biotherapy principle of low-level laser treatment. It uses thirty laser diodes to produce the light laser and rotates around the head 180 degrees, so that it can penetrate the thinnest areas of growth uniformly. The rotational treatment is believed to be more efficient in delivering laser light to the scalp than systems that supply focused energy to one spot at a time and, because it operates automatically, human error is also eliminated from the process. Because hair loss in women is typically diffuse thinning over the entire scalp, rotational phototherapy is theoretically an ideal treatment. Hair growth studies using the Revage system have shown that 85 percent of people receiving treatments with the system have seen hair loss taper off and 39 percent of patients report seeing an increase in fullness. This type of system is only used in doctor's offices or hair clinics. The initial treatment sessions are done twice a week for the first six weeks. It is recommended that touch-up treatments be done periodically to maintain the level of hair growth desired.

Although large laser therapy units have been in use in treatment centers in Europe for more than ten years for a variety of therapeutic uses, including stimulation of hair growth in treatments provided by hair clinics and hair restoration centers, low-level laser devices are now marketed by several companies for at-home use. The differences between the professional and at-home laser units include primarily size and operability, including the novel use of "teeth" in handheld comb-type units that part the hair for treatment. The Lexington HairMax Laser Comb, approved as a device by the FDA in

2007, is designed for use at home. Developed by an Australian company, it was lauded by *Time* magazine as an Invention of the Year for its high-quality ergonomic design. The device complies with safety requirements for U.S. laser products and is patented and manufactured in the United States. Units of this type have all the technical components of the larger laser systems, but are contained in compact units that have comblike teeth to part the hair, allowing laser light to effectively reach more of the scalp areas that need treatment.

The Bernstein Medical Center for Hair Restoration in New York City has developed a proprietary, ergonomically designed handheld laser system that is also designed for home use. Called the X5 Hair Laser, the unit is manufactured by Spencer Forest. This battery-operated unit uses fifteen diodes to provide laser irradiation of the scalp, covering areas over 9 square inches each time it passes over the head. The laser output is slightly more than other small LLLT units, but it's still a low-level unit that's considered entirely safe for home and clinic use. Existing hair growth doesn't interfere with the distribution of the laser light, which is able to make direct contact with the scalp—the major difference between this handheld unit and others on the market. Besides fitting comfortably in the palm of the hand, the system is also cordless, which allows for greater freedom of movement for the user during use. An LCD display on top of the unit shows the user how much time has elapsed in the treatment and indicates how much battery power is left.

Other LLLT models are available for both professional and at-home use. The Aculas Laser, for example, is classified as medical electrical equipment under European CE Certification (EMC Directive 93/94 EEC) and has other medical approvals pending. It is touted by the manufacturer as being "the most powerful home low-level laser therapy to improve the cosmetic appearance of your hair, making it appear thicker, fuller, and healthier." The uniquely designed system is said to offer more direct laser power and laser modules than any competitive unit, with guaranteed electrical safety (CE approval). Three different types of units, including a laser comb, are offered by Aculas, each having a different power supply and pricing that ranges from US$899 to $1,214. Depending on the individual's diagnosis, concomitant use of minoxidil may be recommended in conjunction with using the Aculas Laser system. Aculas products are sold primarily through the Web store Psoriasis Cafe (www.psoriasiscafe.org/aculas.htm). It is not yet approved as a medical device in the United States but can be purchased for cosmetic use.

MAKING HEADWAY IN CLONING HAIR

You have undoubtedly heard about Dolly, the now famous sheep in Scotland who was the first animal ever cloned. It might seem that it would be easier to clone a single hair than to clone a whole sheep, which of course is what cloning is designed to do. However, if we can understand how we got Dolly through the process of cloning, we can possibly understand how, in the future, our own hair could be cloned to replace lost hair as needed. Producing Dolly proved to scientists that nonsex cells, called somatic cells, of a whole adult organism had the potential to develop into an entirely new adult organism of the same type. This was contrary to scientists' earlier thinking that specialized cells such as those of a lung or liver could not become other types of organ cells, since other genes in those cells were inactivated once the organ cell took on the discrete function of the organ. The greatest challenge in cloning was for the scientists to multiply genetically altered cells and then create the perfect environment in which the growth of an entirely new organism could be fostered. Basically, to produce Dolly, the scientists took genetic material—the DNA-containing nucleus of an adult sheep cell designated as the donor—and transferred it into a sheep's egg from which the genetic material had been removed. Now the sheep egg contained DNA from the donor cell instead of its own DNA. Cell division, which occurs biologically and automatically within sheep cells of a single fertilized sheep egg, was stimulated by means of either chemical treatment or an electrical current. At a certain point in its development, the newly cloned sheep embryo was moved into the uterus of another sheep, who "hosted" the clone until it was time for its birth. It doesn't sound like such a complicated process, but that's because we're not getting into the years of theorizing and experimentation by genetic scientists before this successful cloning took place and brought Dolly into the world. Their work has given us a living example of the potential of cloning and has also posed unlimited possibilities—and many controversies as well.

When can we expect hair cloning to happen? There's no way to tell. Research continues. But let's review what we do know about cloning techniques and hair follicles. Scientists are convinced that cloning of hair in the same manner as Dolly was cloned would be impossible because (1) follicles are too complicated to be cloned by culturing them in a test tube, and (2) follicles aren't whole organisms. Although these things are true, experiments by Dr. Reynolds and her colleagues have shed more light on hair cloning and the techniques that could make it possible and someday even commonplace. Scientists know now, for example, that cells from the lower part of the human hair follicle, called the dermal sheath cells, can be taken from one person, isolated, and then injected into another person's skin to create full terminal hair follicles and hair growth. Follicle cells have been taken from a male donor and have been implanted in a female recipient, with full terminal hair growth and no rejection as there might be with other transplanted cells viewed as "foreign" by the immune system. Apparently, the implanted dermal sheath cells from follicles as used in these experiments have an immune system advantage of some kind that precludes rejection. This is a good thing! In addition, the resulting new hair has been found to resemble the recipient's hair, not the donor's. Another good thing! And there's more to be excited about. Even though transferring cells from one person to another is possible, it may not be necessary except in the case of replacing hair in someone who is completely bald. If someone with androgenetic alopecia has hair growing across the sides and back of the head in sufficient quantity, the follicle cells could be obtained from this supply, eliminating the need for another donor. Furthermore, follicle cells can be *multiplied* rather than classically cloned, allowing an unlimited source of donor hairs and production of unlimited numbers of hair follicles through implantation—enough to replace any amount of balding.

There is still much to learn about successful cloning, but it's reassuring to know that scientists are working on it. As it was with Dolly, finding the perfect environment in which cells can grow will make the difference in the results of hair cloning—and will also determine when we see cloning hair as a clinically proven means for hair replacement.

WHAT ELSE IS ON THE HORIZON FOR HAIR?

New drugs are always in development and new indications for existing drugs. Drugs for treating hair loss have not been high on the list of research priorities because, as I said way back in the beginning of the alopecia story, hair loss is not deadly; it does not kill us. Diseases that command attention are the ones with high rates of mortality and morbidity. Hair loss affects our quality of life, but we can survive it, that much is certain. So, given this state of hair affairs, what can we expect from creative researchers that may some day effectively address androgenetic alopecia or other types of alopecia that lead to thinning or balding? Alternatives and future treatment options, except for the grafting of synthetic fibers, are primarily directed toward the cellular level of hair restoration. New types of surgical hair restoration include follicle regeneration and the development of new synthetic donor fibers; and gene technologies such as genetic engineering, discovery of the gene that causes androgenetic alopecia, and hair multiplication. And wouldn't it be great to know that the benefits of all new treatments—new drug therapies included—were indicated for treatment of alopecia in *women*—not only men.

Follicle Regeneration—An Advance in Surgical Hair Restoration

In the hair transplantation arena, much research is being focused on follicle regeneration. Clinical studies have already shown that sectioning a hair follicle horizontally across the perifollicular sheath produces two portions that will each continue to grow. That means that a single follicular unit, when grafted, could logically result in at least two grafts, maybe more. For individual transplant recipients, this could substantially increase the overall availability of donor grafts, allowing many more people to qualify as candidates for hair transplantation. Research is also under way on the possibility of cloning hair follicle stem cells. It's controversial, yes, but could ultimately produce an unlimited supply of donor grafts, virtually revolutionizing surgical hair restoration.

New Materials for Synthetic Hair Grafts

Synthetic hair grafts are not entirely new; they were introduced in Japan in 1972 and are used today in many countries, but not yet in the United States because no clinical studies have demonstrated the safety of synthetic grafts. However, new materials are being explored through clinical research (e.g., by Ethicon, a Johnson & Johnson company in the United States), including polyethylene terephthalate, a material already used medically for suturing wounds, with amorphous silver incorporated as a coating to provide antibacterial activity. Infection and progressive scarring are the most frequent complications of synthetic hair grafts, due primarily to the immune system's reaction to foreign bodies. Another big drawback to be overcome is that the synthetic materials used to date have an unnatural appearance and frequently require replacement to maintain any semblance of real hair. There is much work to be done on this front, and considering the ongoing success of surgical hair transplants using the recipient's own hair follicles, it remains to be seen what the advantages might be of developing new material for synthetic hair grafting. Considering the high costs associated with surgical transplant procedures, price could be a possible advantage when new synthetic fibers finally become available.

Genetic Engineering—A Cousin to Cloning

Genetic engineering is the first thing that comes to mind when we consider the technologies being explored today that might be applied to correcting hair loss. The purpose of genetic engineering, unlike cloning, is to alter the DNA of an individual cell so that it develops specific proteins that can correct genetic defects or possibly improve the functioning or characteristics of the organism in some way. Genes responsible for a particular defect, for example, are isolated and cloned, or multiplied. The modified or altered gene is then placed inside a cell where it is expected to do its work to correct the targeted defect.

Hair Multiplication

Hair multiplication is something quite different from either cloning or genetic engineering—and quite theoretical at the moment. It involves the selective plucking of hairs from the scalp (or sometimes from the beard in men) and implanting them into bald areas. Germinative stem cells at the base of extracted hair follicles are believed to be capable of regenerating new follicles after they are implanted. If this theory holds true, an unlimited supply of hair follicles could be regenerated and permanent hair growth could be encouraged in bald areas of a healthy scalp. A variation of the procedure separates the bulbs of hairs from the shafts and the stem cells are grown *outside* the body, injecting them later into pores of the scalp. The one drawback to either version of the procedure is that stem cells at the base of the follicle that are capable of regenerating a follicle and regrowing hair are not obtained in sufficient quantity through this hair-plucking process. It is a process that requires much more investigation and experimentation, but like cloning and genetic engineering, holds some promise for more effective ways to reproduce a natural head of hair, or at least fill balding spots.

134

Identifying the Gene that Causes Androgenetic Alopecia

We've already learned about androgenetic alopecia, the genetically influenced alopecia that causes pattern hair loss. The gene defect responsible for this has not yet been identified, but it's not because scientists aren't looking. A gene has been identified that causes significant hair loss in infants, and in this condition, the hair that is lost is never replaced. Although this is a rare disease and the gene is not the one responsible for the pattern hair loss that affects millions of men and women, the same scientists, Dr. Amanda Reynolds and Dr. Colin Jahoda, who discovered the gene, are working hard to identify the gene we all want to know about—the one that causes androgenetic alopecia. You can be sure we'll hear the news when *this* gene is identified!

CHAPTER 7

NONSURGICAL HAIR REPLACEMENT AND COSMETIC ENHANCEMENT

Nonsurgical hair replacement products (hair systems, hair weaves, hairpieces), cosmetic hair enhancing products (fibers, topical treatments, hair and scalp treatment systems), other products for hair loss and normal hair care ... and, buyer be wary—are product claims too good to be true?

REPLACING LOST HAIR ... OR ENHANCING HAIR GROWTH

When you first consult a medical professional about alopecia, the topic of hair replacement is mainly about identifying the type of alopecia you have and deciding on the appropriate treatment for it. From that point on, however, hair replacement becomes all about aesthetics—what the final outcome will look like and especially how natural it will look. Determining the reason for hair loss is critical, of course—it's an appropriate first step. The next step, determining what needs to be done to replace your lost hair or encourage hair to grow, is equally important. But asking, "How will it look?" is right up there in terms of important questions!

So, assuming that you've read the previous chapters about medical and surgical treatments, you're now familiar with FDA-approved medications that protect the scalp and/or stimulate the growth of hair, and with surgical hair replacement options and enhanced hair growth with low-level laser. Finally, it's about time for you to get acquainted with modern *nonsurgical* options for hair restoration—or restoring the appearance of your hair with a range of *hair enhancement* options. You will undoubtedly find it helpful to understand the full range of medical, surgical, and cosmetic options in order to decide what's right for you and your particular type of alopecia. The solution could be surgical only, nonsurgical only, or camouflage only—or a thoughtful combination of approaches to get the intended result you want. If you learn as much as you can about all the approaches that are available before you make your decision and act on it, of course you'll feel more satisfied when you know you've made an informed choice. You should also be thinking about the specific result you want. How you want to look has *everything* to do with your product or treatment choices.

IDENTIFYING YOUR AESTHETIC GOALS

Nonsurgical hair replacement or "hair addition" refers to the use of external hair-bearing devices that are either added to existing hair or affixed to the scalp in some way to create the appearance of a full, or fuller, head of hair. Included in these devices are hair weaves, hair extensions, hairpieces, hair prostheses, and wigs.

Cosmetic hair enhancement options vary from camouflage for thinning hair to topical products that promote a healthy scalp and follicles, and some that promise to restore hair growth.

Knowing your aesthetic goals will help you make a decision about nonsurgical or enhancement options that will work best for you considering the type of alopecia you have and the extent of your hair loss or thinning. You can start by asking yourself these questions:

- What hairstyle have I been wearing? Does it conceal hair loss? Is it time to change?
- Is my scalp showing noticeably in places or is my hair thinning all over?
- How much of my hair needs to be restored? What scalp areas?
- After my hair is restored by surgery, growth enhancement, or cosmetic options, what hairstyle would I prefer? Do I need partial or full hair replacement to have this style?
- Do I need a hair replacement that allows me to engage in physical exercise, swimming, or dancing without worrying?
- How thick do I want my hair to appear?
- Do I want my natural hair color matched or is this an opportunity to change it?
- Am I a candidate for transplantation? (See chapter 6.)
- If I'm not a transplant candidate, am I willing to investigate or undergo hair weaving?
- Am I willing to investigate or to wear a partial or complete hairpiece?

- Would I be willing to create the illusion of thicker hair rather than have surgery or wear a hairpiece?
- Do I prefer to hold out for regrowing my own hair rather than to replace hair nonsurgically or camouflage my hair loss?
- Do I have a budget in mind for correcting my hair loss problem? Asked another way: how much am I willing and able to spend?

Once you're satisfied with your own answers, discussing these questions with your doctor or physician hair replacement specialist will help you decide which options would be most apt to give you your desired result. Hair replacement consultants will give you medical, aesthetic, and financial advice to help determine whether surgical or nonsurgical methods, or a combination of the two, will be most appropriate for you and most closely meet your aesthetic goals. Financial goals must be considered, too, of course.

It's also important to consider whether you're looking for a temporary solution or a permanent one. If your hair loss is temporary, for example, as a result of chemotherapy or a reversible underlying disease, then total hair replacement with a prosthesis or wig may provide an effective temporary solution until hair growth resumes. These options can also be a satisfying permanent solution if you have a genetic condition that precludes normal hair growth or if you are not a suitable candidate for transplantation. And remember, if your alopecia has not yet been diagnosed, you're not ready to commit to nonsurgical hair replacement until you know your hair growth status.

BEFORE YOU DECIDE ... BE MINDFUL OF PRODUCT CLAIMS

Hundreds of products are being marketed that claim to treat pattern hair loss or hair thinning from any cause. Claims are not always supported by proof of safety and efficacy; for example, several medications are patented but only topical minoxidil is FDA approved to date and therefore it's a recognized medical treatment (see "About Minoxidil," chapter 5). This chapter will report on a smattering of the different types of products available today—a variety of nonsurgical hair replacement methods and cosmetic hair products that claim to enhance hair growth or enhance the appearance of thinning hair. The idea is to give you an overview of the types of products that are available, not to promote one product over another. To assist you, I've researched these products primarily on the Internet as you will likely do. I've also added a list of Web resources at the back of the book (See "Web sites" in Resources) and also within this chapter. The nonsurgical methods described are all in current use. The claims are the manufacturers' in most cases, sometimes corroborated by clinical studies or expert opinion, and sometimes hyped by the Web store with no corroboration of claims at all. The products are presented just to acquaint you with how many options are open to you. Please remember that I am not recommending any product or manufacturer or verifying any product claims. I urge you to be cautious and to research any products that interest you; and, above all, to consult your doctor before jumping into a treatment program of your own design.

REPLACING LOST OR THINNING HAIR WITH HAIR WEAVES AND HAIR ADDITIONS

The goal of today's hair weaves and hair additions is to give you natural-looking, undetectable weaves and partial or complete hairpieces using natural human hair, synthetic fibers, or a combination of these. Combining different types of treatments may also provide solutions—such as combining the advantages of follicular unit hair grafting techniques (see chapter 6) with the use of hairpieces to achieve more comprehensive coverage, to address a specific pattern of alopecia, or to mask scarring of the scalp. Fortunately, advances in the design of hair additions and improved fixation techniques have given users access to a broad range of natural hairstyles. A hair addition, by the way, is considered to be any external hair-bearing device that when added to your own hair or scalp, gives the appearance of a fuller head of hair. Included under the general heading of additions are hair weaves, hair extensions, hairpieces, toupees, nonsurgical hair replacements, cranial prostheses, partial hair prostheses, hair wefts, and more. Advances in technology have brought these products a long way since your high school principal wore a toupee or your great-aunt covered her see-through hair with a wig that slipped when she sneezed. However, these hair solutions—whether we call them hairpieces, hair systems, extensions, toupees, or wigs—are not just sitting on a shelf waiting for you ... and if they are, you probably won't want them. Today's quality hair additions are almost all custom made for your head only, your hair color and texture, and can be tailored to your individual needs and preferences, including how you want them to attach to your hair or scalp. They are certainly a lot less expensive initially than hair transplantation procedures. However, except for certain hair weaving techniques, they need replacing every so often (from 4 to 6 times a year, depending on the type and the material), which increases their cost over a period of years, whereas transplants can last a lifetime. The decision is entirely yours and is based on the result you want. You'll need to rely on the guidance of a hair restoration specialist to make sure that your individual hair replacement and aesthetic needs are met.

Hair Weaves

Hair weaving is a hair-to-hair replacement procedure, in contrast to hair-to-scalp replacement. The most notable use of hair weaving in the United States was introduced by Hair Club for Men over thirty years ago. No longer just providing treatment for men, the club has been renamed and registered Hair Club and has redirected its promotion and services to men and women. The company's approach, it says, is "about more"—not only in what they offer ("more solutions, more answers, more possibilities") but in what you have to gain. After perusing their material online (www.hairclub.com), I'm inclined to agree. The only problem I have with Hair Club information is that surgical transplantation and other trusted surgeries are criticized as being outdated, without giving recognition to advances in recent years. This does not detract, however, from the offerings of the Hair Club. I recommend that you read their material carefully—it's not all presented in depth (e.g., two paragraphs on the causes of hair loss in women)—and speak to a physician hair restoration specialist who works with the company before you come to any conclusions or make a decision. They do have a lot to offer (including transplant procedures as well as weaves) and you need to know specifically what they can offer you.

The original Hair Club process is patented and has been refined over the years so that men and women who undergo treatment are generally satisfied with the level of restoration cosmetically. Hair weaves are strictly cosmetic and do not correct the underlying hair loss problem—and promotion of the Hair Club product has never made these claims. Here's how it works. Hair weaving techniques create a woven crisscross of transparent hair fibers to form a matrix (the patented Hair Club "BioMatrix" Strand-by Strand process) that is specially fitted and shaped to each client's balding area. The matrix is further developed by gradually weaving in new hairs a strand at a time, following the client's own hair pattern and flow. Using a medical adhesive called Polyfuse, the matrix is finally fused to the growing hair that remains on the head. Once applied, the matrix remains porous, which permits the scalp to breathe as it normally would. New hair can be added to the matrix and hairs can be cut or trimmed as any normal head of hair would be. Clients return to Hair Club stylists about once a month to get haircuts and to have the adhesive replaced. People who have completed the process are very satisfied and, when asked, freely state that they think of it as their own hair and not remotely as a wig or hairpiece.

Hair weaving may have started at a men's hair club, but hair weaves are finally becoming more popular among women, especially postmenopausal women whose hair has begun to thin naturally (female AGA) or who have had an underlying health problem that has resulted in thinning hair or who are taking a drug that causes hair loss. Whatever the reason, hair weaving can provide a happy solution—and a fairly immediate solution. Your hair looks thicker instantly. The process can be tedious but a good result is worth your investment in time and patience. And the weave, if well done, will essentially be invisible. Yes, regular maintenance will be needed, but we're used to maintaining our own hair and maintaining your weave will not be much different. It's matter of priorities!

Hair Extensions

Hair extensions are in the public eye all the time, although we don't always know we're looking at them. You may see an actress in a movie with a shockingly short haircut and see her again in a week or two at the Academy Award ceremonies, as a guest on *Ellen*, or a spot on *Entertainment Tonight* and she has long hair piled up and hanging down her back. We couldn't grow hair that fast even before we experienced thinning. How do they do it? Hair extensions. And you can do it too—adding more hair to your own hair in an attractive "do." No one will know but you.

Some hair extensions clip on and others are woven onto existing hair, but the first step is always carefully matching color and texture. Clip-on extensions must be compatible with your style as well; and you will need to learn from your stylist or extension expert how to fasten the extension to your own hair in a stable way to create the most desirable hairstyle.

Extensions that are woven into your hair are also first matched to your own hair for the closest color and texture. In the attachment process, several pieces of hair are bonded to yours at the scalp level, not unlike the weaving process described above but without creating a matrix. Not surprisingly, human hair extensions are more expensive than synthetic extensions and do provide a more natural appearance.

Adhesives provide another way for extensions to be fastened to your hair. These extensions (wefts) are prepared ahead of time, already bonded together at one end using an adhesive. When they are added to your hair, the end with the adhesive is joined to your hair at the scalp (hair to hair, not hair to scalp) using either a heating method or an ultrasound technique. Is this type of extension safe and durable? People who have had extensions added to their hair will say yes or no, depending on their own experience. Choosing the salon or hair replacement expert who will apply your extension involves a carefully considered personal decision—and it can make all the difference in how you will answer the "safe and durable" question.

It's important to note that the safety of adhesives has improved whether we're talking about double-faced tape or the newest waterproof liquids used with extensions. Most are promoted as being safe by the manufacturers and good results have been reported by extension users. However, be sure to have a patch test done by a dermatologist before applying a hair extension with adhesive, particularly if you have allergies of any kind.

One caution with extensions is that you are adding weight to your own hair when you add a woven extension, and this may create tension on the hair shaft and stress on follicles, especially with hair that's already thinning. The result can be traction alopecia (see "Traction Alopecia," chapter 3), and you're right back to where you started. If your hair is already thin, woven extensions may not be the choice for you. Take the time to research the salons or hair clinics near you (www.ahlc.org or www.hairextensions.com) where extensions are applied and make sure your "expert" has plenty of experience and good results. It's all right to ask how many procedures the stylist has done and to ask for references and even for photographs of satisfied clients. Has this operator or stylist been trained by the hair extension manufacturer? Find out first. This is your head; you want the best result and that will take a quality hair product and the best person you can find to attach your extension and care for it thereafter.

Hairpieces

Hairpieces are either premade or custom designed to cover thinning or balding areas on the scalp. They are made of human hair or synthetic fibers or a combination of the two. They can provide partial cover-up or full coverage and affix to the scalp with double-faced adhesive tapes or liquid adhesives—no more lost or slipping hairpieces. You will have to give your hairpiece the same care you give your own hair—regular washing, conditioning, and styling. And replacement is a given; the hairpiece will fade and lose its fit over time.

Hair Prostheses and Wigs

Prostheses and wigs—they sound like the same thing, don't they? And essentially they are. Both prostheses and wigs are externally worn, artificial hairpieces—full heads of hair designed to cover your *entire* head. The difference is that hair prostheses or *cranial prostheses*, sometimes referred to crassly as "cancer wigs," are handcrafted on a hypoallergenic cranial mold of an individual's head, duplicating the unique shape and contour of the head and resulting in a fit as close as a second skin. Human hair is then sewn into this precisely fitted cap, creating the most natural appearance of growth and flow of hair. The color of the sewn-in human hairs can be uniform throughout or blended to create a distinctive natural color. Individual styling completes the prosthesis.

A wig can also be tailor made, although the majority of wigs are premade by sewing real or synthetic hair to a caplike base that is fitted to the head. The cap is generally constructed of smooth elastic webbing or a woven material that can stretch to achieve a closer fit to the head. Hair is sewn into this webbing by machine—either human hair or synthetic fibers—and the final result is virtually undetectable as a wig and perfectly comfortable because of the airflow allowed by the webbing. Unless it is custom made, the wig is prestyled when you buy it. It will need periodic cleaning and styling, which is not done while you wear it but with the wig removed. Hair integration is similar to having a wig, but the underlying webbing is constructed very loosely so that your own hair can be combed through it. The result is extremely natural but color matching becomes more important because of the combination of your own hair and human hair sewn onto the webbing. Integration is a technique that works best when you just want to add thickness to your hair.

The biggest difference between cranial prostheses and wigs has to do with insurance coverage. Prostheses are ordered by physicians for patients who have lost significant amounts of hair through medical treatment such as chemotherapy (anagen effluvium) or because they have been diagnosed with alopecia areata or trichotillomania. "Full cranial hair prosthesis" is the terminology that must be used when the patient applies for medical insurance coverage. Seeking coverage from your medical insurance plan for a wig will result in being turned down. However, insurance companies are well aware, or are becoming more aware, that alopecia and cancer-related hair loss are justifiable reasons for needing a cranial prosthesis. It must be prescribed by your physician, who can provide all the proper information to justify your claim. A letter from you explaining your situation, and even a photograph of you to show your hair loss, can accompany the claim form as supportive information.

Both prostheses and wigs become part of you and, as such, become part of your regular hygiene and beauty regimen. They can last a long time, depending on your lifestyle, the type of activities you participate in, the nature of your work, and the care you're willing to give. The degree of quality in the full-coverage wig or prosthesis will be noticeable to you. The highest quality pieces and the most natural results are achieved with human hair hand-tied to a custom-made cap. They are also the most expensive.

Preparing for the Costs of Nonsurgical Hair Replacement

Hairpieces and surgical transplants can produce acceptable cosmetic results for all forms of alopecia, but you need to consider, first of all, that these are generally expensive treatments. Actual costs can be obtained from the source of the procedure, device, or replacement system, but it's good to understand ahead of time that procedures and devices considered nonmedical or "cosmetic" are not covered by standard medical insurance policies. Your costs will be out of pocket and will vary depending on whether the products or services are provided by a physician such as a cosmetic dermatologist, a hair replacement center, or a cosmetologist specializing in hair products, or even the manufacturer of products such as those offered on the Internet. Custom-made hairpieces are viewed as more natural and aesthetically pleasing than off-the-shelf products, a fact that is reflected in their comparative costs. Materials will affect costs as well; human hair products are generally more expensive than synthetic products, for example. When making a decision about hair replacement, it's important to consider replacement costs as well as the initial cost of a hairpiece or replacement device, since hair additions, color and styling can begin to change after eighteen months of wear, so it is not unrealistic to expect to replace a hair addition or wig about every two years. Regular care for a hairpiece, including cleaning, is another financial consideration. Hair transplantation is more expensive initially, but the result is permanent, and a side-by-side cost comparison with long-term nonsurgical solutions may surprise you. Be sure to weigh it out before deciding. And remember, too, that even if you start out with a nonsurgical approach, you can decide at any time to have a transplant, as long as you meet the requirements (see chapter 6).

COSMETIC HAIR ENHANCEMENT PRODUCTS—
FROM CAMOUFLAGE TO FOLLICLE TREATMENT

Dozens of products are available that claim to create the appearance of thicker hair. Dozens more include topical treatments that claim to help maintain a healthy scalp and follicles, thereby encouraging the regrowth of hair. Not all of these products are described as able to regrow hair, but the implication seems to be that restoring the health of follicles will *help* to regrow hair. First, it actually does sound entirely believable that if the scalp is not scarred, then follicles can be restimulated to work as intended, and secondly, we know that hair growth is the product of working follicles. However, actual end results are determined case by case. Only your doctor or cosmetic dermatologist can tell you what your chances are of successfully regrowing hair after treatment for your type of alopecia.

One type of hair-thickening product consists of synthetic hairlike fibers that are applied in some fashion to the scalp or to other hairs. Other enhancement products are applied topically with the intended result of camouflaging areas of the scalp that have lost hair; still others are topical treatment systems of various types, making different claims about enhancing the appearance of hair and/or improving the health of follicles to ultimately stimulate hair growth. There are even products that claim to *prevent* hair loss if androgenetic alopecia is the diagnosis. All of these products are in the *cosmetic* category; none is considered to be a *medical* product, although some that are described as DHT inhibitors may contain clinically tested and approved medications for hair loss such as minoxidil and aminexil. Certain products have not been studied or approved in the United States, or are approved only as cosmetic

145

products, and for this reason I have included them here rather than discussing them in the earlier chapter on medical treatments.

I describe one or two of each type of cosmetic enhancement product here (without having tried them myself, please note) and give you the names and contact information of suppliers or manufacturers so that you can investigate the products on your own and find the one or ones that suit you best. To be sure, many more products can be found on the Internet than those included here; my intent is only to present a variety of options. Once you understand the comprehensive range of products available, and the various categories of hair enhancement techniques, you'll be able to research products or categories on the Internet and get a good sense of which ones you might be willing to try.

The claims sometimes seem too good to be true, so be sure you investigate products well before you buy, not only because they can be expensive, but they generally don't come with guarantees.

Nevertheless, be assured—there is absolutely a solution for you. Again, it all depends on your aesthetic goals and the ultimate result you want.

Consult the Resources section at the back of this book to find out more about Internet sources and Web stores that offer a full range of nonsurgical hair replacement and hair enhancement products.

Fiber Products

Fiber products are becoming increasingly popular because they are designed to blend with your own hair and create the appearance of a thicker, fuller head of hair almost instantly. Consisting of tiny, microfiber "hairs," these products are not merely cover-ups—the fibers physically intertwine with thin velluslike hairs on your own head to literally make them thicker. The organic fibers used in these products are derived from the naturally occurring keratin in sheep wool, the very same type of keratin protein that is present in your own hair. Static electricity helps them bond to your hair, keeping the fibers interwoven and in place as you go about your daily activities. Users say that they even withstand a night's sleep. Fiber products are reported to produce an instant result. They are prepared in containers that allow you to shake on the microfibers over the thinning parts of your scalp, spreading thousands of tiny hair fibers into your own hair on a single application. In several products, the fibers are described as coming in eight colors so they can be closely color-matched to your own hair color. Users report that they can't see the fibers no matter how closely they look for them—even immediately after applying them. Fibers can be used alone as a hair thickener, or can be used in conjunction with hair-growth products like minoxidil to help hide balding areas that are beginning to regrow hair. Users, many of whom are middle-aged women with female pattern baldness, consider fibers to be "amazing" and "magic." They report that the fiber product is not just hair enhancing, but life enhancing. "Nanogen has given me the confidence to meet challenges head on," said one happy user, explaining further, "like traveling for work and meeting lots of people." Nanogen Electrostatic Fibers is a fiber product manufactured in Europe; it's available in the United States through the salon Web store www .onlyhairloss.com. More detailed information about fibers and other products is also available on that site. Another fiber product manufactured in the United States, Toppik Hair Building Fibers, is manufactured by Spencer Forrest Labs in Westport, Connecticut (800-416-3325; www.toppik.com/ toppik.asp).

Topical Creams, Lotions, and Gels

Grooming aids of all kinds are used by men and women for better-looking hair. It's not unusual, therefore, to find that applying creams, lotions, or gels to the hair to promote hair growth or to mask thinning or balding areas of the scalp is appealing to those who seek these benefits. Convenient packaging and special applicators are common accessories and many have companion products such as shampoos and nutritional supplements in a topical form. Couvré by AMSG Enterprises is one such product, and can be found on Dr. Robert Bernstein's informative site (www .BernsteinMedical.com.) as well as www.afountainofyouth.net, a site that discusses and sells many hair loss remedies. The manufacturer claims that the lotion compound eliminates the contrast between your hair and scalp, making balding patches look fuller and thinning areas disappear altogether. Couvré lotion is sold with Couvré Thickening Shampoo and Couvré Protein Hair Expander. The shampoo is reported to volumize the hair and to remove the harmful buildup of sebum that makes hair appear limp. The hair-expanding product has a high concentration of organic proteins that penetrate the exterior of the hair shaft to deliver the proteins into the hair and make it appear thicker. The Couvré products are designed to be used together.

Sprays and Powders

Thinning hair may not require replacing per se, but it can benefit from cosmetic thickening to give the appearance of a fuller head of hair and to help mask minor balding spots. Colored hair-thickening sprays or non colored aerosol hair-thickening spray-on systems can quite easily add texture and volume to thinning hair. Some contain thickening resin that is resistant to rubbing and water. Although these products don't eliminate bald spots, they cosmetically reduce the appearance of bald spots, especially on the crown of the head or along the part. Sprays stay in until you shampoo them out. Fullmore, manufactured by Spencer Forrest Labs (800-416-3325; www.toppik.com), is an example of a colored hair-thickening spray; ProThik is a water-resistant aerosol spray-on system (800-710-8445; www.prothik.com).

Hair for 2 (Volluma) is a spray that is said to "attach itself to hair," clinging firmly to each hair to make individual hairs stronger and the head of hair to appear thicker and stronger. The spray is said to be totally invisible and even from an inch away, it is impossible to see that someone has used the product. The manufacturer says it is totally invisible and is resistant to rain and normal perspiration. It is recommended for use with minoxidil or aminexil, a minoxidil-like product, or after hair transplantation, as long as the scalp is completely healed. Information about Hair for 2 can be found at www.hairloss-hair-loss.com/hairloss/volluma.htm.

Powder cakes offer another cosmetic approach, featuring a hard-packed powder that both coats and colors thin hairs. When applied with a wet sponge applicator, the powder coating instantly creates the appearance of thicker hair and helps to mask bald spots by coloring the scalp beneath thinning areas. The powdered cosmetic coats each hair so that it stands up and spreads out, creating overall fullness when an entire area is treated. The product also conditions hair and moisturizes the scalp. Treated hair can be brushed. Derm-Match, Inc., in Venice, Florida, manufactures DermMatch Powder Cake and other hair products (800-826-2824; www.dermatch.com).

DHT Inhibitors or Blockers

You learned earlier in this book that an enzyme called 5-alpha-reductase converts the body's natural testosterone into a more potent androgen, called DHT, that can be present at high levels in hair follicles and in the scalp of some individuals—both men and women who have signs of pattern baldness.

DHT is one of the causes of pattern baldness, and inhibitors of DHT are used to encourage follicle health and normal hair growth. Minoxidil, which is described in detail in chapter 5, is a recognized DHT inhibitor that has been approved by the FDA for use in the United States as a hair growth stimulant. Rogaine, the trade name for the minoxidil product introduced by Merck, is the leading minoxidil product, but others are available.

One such product being promoted is actually a complete system for hair growth, including 5 percent minoxidil, shampoo-in nutritional supplements, a topical spray that increases blood flow to the scalp, and a scalp cleanser that unclogs pores. The system is described by the manufacturer as able to combat "all of the major causes of hair loss," namely, decreased scalp circulation, the DHT effect on follicles, lack of essential nutrients for hair growth, and presence of harmful microbes in clogged pores. This patented product is Follicare Hair Growth and Restoration System, a trademark of Advanced BodyCare Solutions, LLC (www.follicare.com).

Aminexil, a European product that works in a similar manner as minoxidil, has been investigated in one clinical study conducted in 1994 to 1995 in various hospitals in Europe and the United States by dermatologist Hans Boerma, M.D. and a team of clinical investigators. (I could not access the published report of this particular study.) The product works by acting on hair follicles to discourage the effects of DHT, rather than directly inhibiting DHT production. Essentially, it is believed to encourage more follicles to be in the anagen phase at any given time, which theoretically would result in more hair growth. Reportedly, results of the clinical study showed that the 130 test participants between the ages of 18 and 55 years who were treated daily with an aminexil shampoo manufactured by Kérastase all had new hair growth when compared to control subjects who used a placebo product. Hair thickness was reported to increase by 6 percent after six weeks of topical applications. The recommended dosage is suggested to be continued for six months or twice a year for six weeks at a time, to sustain continued growth in individuals, both men and women, with androgenetic alopecia. The product is recommended also for seasonal hair loss or to correct overall thinning. Aminexil has a global patent. More information is available at www.hairloss-hair-loss.com/hairloss/aminexil_results.htm. I describe aminexil here rather than in the chapter on medical treatment, because clinical information is not readily available in online medical resources and the product is not approved by the FDA for use in the United States.

Growth serums have been developed and marketed by other companies as well. Asia and Europe seem to be way ahead of North America in developing and promoting hair loss therapies that are reported to work by developers, physicians, and users. Part of the reason, besides centuries-old acceptance in Asian and European countries of using botanicals for treating various conditions, is that the approval process in countries outside the United States is generally less stringent and also faster, allowing products to be tested, marketed, and used almost simultaneously. A hair growth serum that includes DHT inhibitors is MegaTHIK Hair Growth Serum, which is said to reduce high levels of DHT, increase circulation to the scalp, and provide vital nutrients to hair follicles. The result of rubbing in this topical scalp treatment, according to the manufacturer, is to thicken and strength hair growth. MegaTHIK is reported to be safe, nonirritating, and able to revitalize the hair of men and women with pattern baldness and overall thinning. Ingredients obtained from Europe and Asia include proteins; hydrogenated castor oil; apigenin; oleanic acid; PEG-40 and PEG-8 dimethicone; the nutrients biotin, panthenol, and zinc; and the herbs nettle and saw palmetto. MegaTHIK is sold in the United States through the salon Web store www.onlyhairloss.com.

NuGen Hp claims to be an all natural two-step treatment for hair loss, one step of which is anti-DHT therapy. The primary NuGen product, NuGen Follicle Enhancer, is described as being able to balance the enzyme 5-alpha-reductase that increases the production of DHT, the hormone responsible for hair thinning in androgenetic alopecia. Use of the phrase "all natural" indicates an herbal or other natural source of anti-DHT as the primary ingredient. Although I was not able to confirm that minoxidil or aminexil is the primary ingredient in NuGen Hp Follicle Enhancer, its intended therapeutic effect is similar. The companion product NuGen Turbo Accelerator uses transdermal delivery via the inside of the wrist to deliver nutrients necessary for hair growth, claiming to produce "thicker, fuller, healthier hair." The term *transdermal*, by the way, simply means "through the skin." Scientific researchers have long known that skin is an ideal delivery system for drugs and other substances. We have seen transdermal delivery at work in skin patches that administer, for example, nitroglycerine to cardiac patients, nicotine to people working on their smoking habit, and hormones for women practicing birth control. In similar fashion, the wrist could be the site of transdermal delivery of nutrients, and the scalp itself becomes a logical delivery system for treating follicles—the source of our hair growth and the source of alopecia in many cases. As we have seen, scientists have developed a broad range of products delivered through the scalp to treat the scalp directly and follicles ultimately—all of them designed to benefit the hair. The NuGen system is intended for use by men or women with thinning hair, not those who are partially or completely bald. Product information states that the FDA has acknowledged the safety of the system. More information is available at www.onlyhairloss .com/nugen_hp; articles and product literature can also be found by searching NuGen Hp Turbo Accelerator.

Another botanical system that claims to inhibit 5-alpha-reductase is offered on hair salon Web stores and supported by a study published in a peer-reviewed journal, *The Journal of Alternative and Complementary Medicine* (vol. 2, 2002). The study demonstrated the effectiveness of the botanically derived ingredients of Hair Genesis in treating androgenetic alopecia. However, the twenty-six participants in the study were all men, which doesn't indicate the effectiveness of the product for women. The product is manufactured by Advanced Restoration Technologies, Inc., in Denver, Colorado (www.hairgenesis.com). More information about the product and the complete scientific study can be found at www.onlyhairloss.com.

Hair Growth Stimulants and Nutrients

Because nearly everyone uses shampoo regularly, it provides a useful delivery system for various ingredients that are described as "hair growth stimulants." Products of this type claim to introduce their ingredients directly into the scalp to not only cleanse the hair and scalp but to provide, among other things, anti-inflammatory action, anti-DHT activity, antioxidant protection against infection, increased scalp vitality, increased size of the hair shaft, and hair growth stimulants.

One of these shampoos is Revita, which contains, according to its manufacturer, the highest research grade of minoxidil. The only other clinically proven medication, they say, is aminexil, a product manufactured in the Netherlands and used as a companion product to Revita, the DHT inhibitor Spectral DNC. Revita and Spectral DNC are manufactured by DSLaboratories (www.hairloss-hair-loss.com/hairloss/aminexil_results.htm), which refers to its proprietary anti-DHT shampoo as an "intelligent cosmetic."

DSL suggests that Revita Shampoo works on its own to protect hair follicles and is also designed to prepare the scalp and hair follicles for treatment with Spectral DNC (the main ingredient is Aminexil SP94). The shampoo is recommended for individuals who have only slight hair loss or are just beginning to lose their hair and, when used as recommended with Spectral DNC, the combo is said to "provide maximum results." The reason given for this success is that it's much easier to prevent hair loss than it is to grow new hair. This being said, it appears that *prevention* of hair loss will be the goal of the ideal candidate for this product. However, it will be necessary to first know the cause of your hair loss before trying this product; Revita and other hair growth stimulants are intended for women (and men) who lose hair as a result of androgenetic alopecia, the same genetically caused alopecia that produces most of the balding seen in men. We've learned that estrogen helps to protect women's hair follicles somewhat from the destructive effects of DHT, but we also know that estrogen levels can go up and down at different times in a woman's life and hair thinning can develop if the genetic susceptibility is present. In this case, Revita appears to be a product that can help protect hair follicles from DHT and help to maintain a fuller head of healthier hair. The makers of Revita claim that it does not cross-react with other topical treatments so you can use it with other products. Again, it would be wise to consult with your doctor before using the product.

Allure magazine named Osmotics FNS Follicle Nutrient Serum a Breakthrough Product of the Year in 2006 for its contribution to treating hair loss in men and women. Not just a single product, Osmotics FNS is described as an "Anti-Aging Hair System for Women," claiming to provide proper nourishment for stress-related hair loss and hereditary hair thinning (androgenetic alopecia or female pattern hair loss). The Osmotics FNS System also includes companion products, including a revitalizing shampoo especially for women and a revitalizing conditioner. As with other systems, Osmotics FNS literature recommends using all of the complementary products to achieve the best hair growth or hair thickening results. The manufacturer says the products also benefit chemically treated or damaged hair. More information is available at Hair Remedies, www.afountainofyouth.net or www.onlyhairloss.com.

Shen Min, a product line derived from Chinese herbs and manufactured in China, claims to have integrated traditional Chinese medicine with modern science to develop their products and describes their hair loss treatment as a "breakthrough" able to achieve full, lustrous, and healthy hair. The product was designed especially for women, but it is said to work equally well for men. Although the ingredients are primarily herbal, the scientific advantage is a natural vine-grown herb, called *fo-ti* or *he-shou wu*, that has been used for centuries in China to turn graying hair back to its natural color. The other herbs are noted for properties such as energizing follicular growth to overcome the changes caused by DHT, the hormone that reduces follicular activity in androgenetic alopecia. The primary product is Advanced Shen Min for Women. Its companion products are Shen Min Activator, Shen Min Nutrient, Shen Min Vitalize Shampoo, and Shen Min Volumizing Serum. Users from Asia, the United States, and Australia all report thicker, more youthful hair and restored color as well as restored hair growth after experiencing losses. They describe seeing results in two to three months. More details about Shen Min products, including how to order, are available at www.onlyhairloss.com/women/shenmin/ about.htm.

Viviscal Nourishment for the Hair, Viviscal Shampoo, and Viviscal Conditioner are designed, according to the manufacturer, to work together "to replace and reenergize nutrients needed for hair growth." The goal of the Viviscal system of products, beginning with the Viviscal concentrated nutrient lotion, is to increase the growth rate of hair and retard thinning. It is described as helping to remove internal barriers that block the flow of nutrients to the scalp, along with hydrating and rejuvenating the scalp. It also allows vitamins and nutrients to pass through the scalp into the hair itself. "Hair grows from the inside out," they say, "and this is why Viviscal was created." More information on this product line and other nutrient-based systems is available at www.afountainofyouth.net/category/1322242541/1/VIVISCAL.htm.

HERBAL SUPPLEMENT THAT CLAIMS TO PROMOTE HAIR GROWTH

Certain herbs or combinations of herbs and botanicals are reported in scientific studies conducted in the Netherlands to have DHT blocking effects when taken orally or used topically, proving to promote hair growth by either route. Unlike finasteride (Propecia) the product has been shown in studies overseas (www.hairloss-hair-loss.com/hairloss/capiplus_ingredients. htm) to be safe for women (with the warning that it should absolutely not be taken by women who are pregnant) and has been shown to grow new

153

hair effectively, as well as to stimulate the hair growth process by supporting hair follicle health and maintaining suppleness of collagen in hair. Capiplus Female, a product advertised "for hereditary hair loss in females and to stimulate new hair growth" has been created by Machi, a company located in the Netherlands. The organic ingredients in Capiplus Female include angelica (the Chinese herb *dong quai*, a women's tonic used for gynecologic conditions and complaints such as PMS and hormone balancing), polygonum multiflorum (an anti-androgen, DHT blocker); the herbs achyranthes, dioscorea, and salvia; vitamins B and C; and minerals zinc and calcium. Minimum duration of use for effective growth of hair is purported to be six months, taking four capsules daily. The herbal supplement can be taken in conjunction with aminexil, the minoxidil-like product widely used in Europe. Machi sells hair products worldwide through the Web store HB Hair Shop (www.hbhairshop .nl; phone 31 (0)651048848). HB, you may be interested to know, stands for Hans Bolder, whose well-known hair salons are based in the Netherlands and who works with L'Oréal Group salons in other European countries.

An important reminder about any of the products discussed here is that I have reported claims by manufacturers or Web sites selling their products. The products are not approved for use in the United States except for some classified as "cosmetic" products, which is the rationale for showing them here, even though they may be considered by the manufacturer to be nutritionally based or may be combined with DHT-inhibiting medication.

CORRECTING HAIR LOSS VIA THE IMMUNE SYSTEM

A most unusual product derived from the thymus gland of calves was originally developed for hair loss prevention in cancer patients receiving chemotherapy. The thymus gland, in cattle as in humans, secretes thymus peptides into the bloodstream to regulate the immune system and its production of antibodies to fight disease. As such, it seemed to be a logical source of protection for follicles during exposure to chemotherapeutic agents that destroy cells. German scientists developed a thymus-based product and clinical studies were conducted in Europe on a large group of cancer patients undergoing chemotherapy. During the course of the study, the product being tested was applied to the scalp of patients prior to their chemotherapy treatments. The results of the study showed that little or no hair fallout occurred, keeping hair loss to a minimum in all patients who participated. After the product was approved for use in Germany, physicians in other countries quickly found out that it also worked for other types of hair loss and scalp disorders, including some of the rare forms of alopecia. The product was soon declared an effective treatment for the regrowth of hair and has since been reported as effective for 67 percent of men who use it and for 95 percent of women. The only requirement is that the follicles of the user must be intact. The formulation of ThymuSkin brand of this effective topical thymus gland product has now been approved by the FDA for cosmetic use in the United States. Studies conducted in the United States have concluded that ThymuSkin indeed stimulates the human immune system, providing increased resistance to infection, cancer, and age-related degenerative disease. Besides boosting the immune system, massaging ThymuSkin into the scalp has been shown to protect hair against fallout and to regrow hair when losses have already occurred. More information is available at www.onlyhairloss.com/thymuskin/about.htm.

COMMONLY USED HAIR CARE PRODUCTS ... SAFE OR NOT?

Whether you use salon brands or brands from the pharmacy or supermarket, certain products are touted as being good for your hair, and others you might want to avoid regardless of claims. Remembering a few tips about these products can help prevent damage.

Detangling combs can be damaging when used on wet hair—which is hair that has been stretched by water—even though operators in the best salons may use them to comb through overprocessed or tangled hair, without giving a thought to the underlying chemistry. Wet hair should never be brushed, period.

Matching the pH—acid versus alkaline—of your hair to your shampoo is important. Salon brand shampoos usually have an acid pH of about 4.5 to 5.5, which is best for your hair because it's familiar to your body. We are acidic animals, for the most part, and acidic shampoos are much like our other body fluids and our skin. Gentle cleansers are also important—harsh detergents will be more alkaline and will remove more of the hair's natural oils, drying hair entirely too much and dulling its sheen.

Conditioners coat hair, relax tangles, and encourage smoother combing as well as extra shine when hair has been dried and styled. Acidic conditioners shrink the outer cuticle and increase alpha bonds in the hair to detangle and add body and shine. Meanwhile, we have to remember our hair chemistry and what happens when we damage cuticles with too many treatments like permanents or coloring—and why we use conditioners to correct these problems. Chemical treatments cause the hairs' cell layers to rise up, exposing the under layers of the cortex, which releases natural moisture and dries out the hair—sometimes severely. When this happens, the raised cells of multiple hairs will grab onto each other, producing the "frizz" and tangles we need to get rid of.

Sun and ultraviolet rays of tanning booths can damage the cuticle of the hair, resulting in frizz and dryness. Shampoos and conditioners are available with sunscreen but even better protection is to cover the head if you're going to be in sunlight for any length of time. And this is not even touching on the problem of a sunburned scalp, which can wreak havoc on hair follicles. It's critical that you use good judgment when exposing your scalp to the sun or the rays of tanning booths.

HAIR MYTHOLOGY—MISTAKEN IDEAS SOMEWHAT ROOTED IN FACT

A range of hair stories can raise the eyebrows of hair care experts who know what's true and what's not when it comes to how hair responds to products and practices. I think it's worthwhile discussing these stories here because these myths often encourage people to diagnose and treat their own hair problems—real or imagined—and risk doing real damage to their hair or scalp. Becoming aware of what's true and not true about hair can help women understand that a hair problem may be more complicated than an everyday hair care issue or something they've caused themselves such as overprocessing of hair with permanent waves, heat, sun, or frequent coloring. The most popular myths or stories, with some expert opinions from Karen Van Wagner at hairfinder.com, and Damien von Dahlem at hair-styles.org, include:

- *The story:* Cutting your hair actually makes it grow faster and become thicker.
  The truth: Cutting hair makes it shorter—period. Any effects of trimming, cutting, or shaving hair are illusions based on the appearance of healthier hair after split ends or shaggy styles are trimmed up. The rate of hair growth is determined by genetics

and health status. Diet can improve your hair growth and appearance more readily than cutting your hair.

- *The story:* Shampooing your hair every day is too much and can dry out your hair.
  The truth: If you're using a shampoo that is right for your hair type and does not contain harsh, potentially drying or damaging detergents and other chemicals, there's nothing to worry about. However, shampooing every other day using a mild shampoo may be a better approach than washing already dry, nonoily hair every day. Daily washing is a waste of shampoo unless your hair or scalp is especially oily. Spend good money on a good shampoo for your type of hair and use less—a more sensible hair policy. If your hair is abnormally dry, consult a dermatologist or a knowledgeable hair salon. Your diet may need adjustment—or a chemical effect received from hair products or treatments may need correcting and the experts know how to do that.

- *The story:* Overstyling can damage hair and cause hair loss.
  The truth: Some styling methods can truly damage hair, causing individual hairs to break off or creating frizz that may need a special treatment to relax the hair shaft. This damage is usually short lived and corrects itself as long as damaged hairs are replaced through a normal hair growth cycle. The only processing that can lead to hair loss, however, is a process that damages follicles. Processes shown to damage follicles include pulling hair tightly into braids and ponytails, or weaving hair into cornrows. This type of follicle damage with associated hair loss is called traction alopecia, traumatic alopecia, or cosmetic alopecia, all referring to the same hairstyle-induced condition.

- *The story:* Hair products should be alternated instead of using the same ones all the time.
  The truth: Hair is not influenced by the same "immunity" that governs cells of the body. Hair does not develop resistance against products but can become coated by certain products, especially conditioners that leave a residue on the hairs. Residues can be removed by using certain clarifying shampoos, by obtaining professional citrus or enzyme treatments, or by rinsing with lemon juice or apple cider vinegar in water.

- ***The story:*** Brushing hair too much can cause it to fall out.
  The truth: Although vigorous brushing can break hairs and result in split ends, gentle brushing with a quality brush should not cause significant hair loss or thin the hair. It's important to note, however, that brushing is actually not necessary for your hair. Regular grooming with a good comb is all that it needs, especially after washing, which actually stretches the hair and requires gentle combing and never brushing. Split ends, by the way, cannot be repaired and should be cut off. Hair loss is an entirely different phenomenon with a range of more complicated causes and explanations—a dermatological problem, not a hair problem.

BUYER BE WARY

At the beginning of chapter 5, I talked about the inventiveness that hair loss has inspired from ancient times until today—starting with bee pollen and bird droppings and progressing to complex nutrient systems. At any given time it seems that opportunists are developing products right along with sincere scientists, both responding to the knowledge that hair loss is a fact of life, and that thinning or balding of any kind is unacceptable. As a result, many products are available that make claims to restore lost hair in record time or to miraculously "grow" or "regrow" hair. Not all of these products and their manufacturers are necessarily focused on any particular type of hair loss or appropriate treatment; sometimes the entire product positioning is based on satisfying cosmetic concerns, not addressing a medical concern.

For example, a wide range of cosmetic products are advertised to "volumize" hair and make it appear thicker, encourage normal hair growth by taking supplements, or to actually grow hair with the topical application of solutions and creams. Advertisers promote a host of theories about hair loss, often clumping all types of hair loss into one catch-all category. The number and claims of products increase continuously—and so do the costs for these products. What are we to do and who are we to believe?

With just one simple Google search for "hair loss," we can see what we're up against. The Internet is a perfect arena for marketing hair loss products and services to unsuspecting individuals who have a real hair loss problem. There are blogs by other hair loss sufferers, Web stores that sell a host of products all directed toward hair care or hair loss, and manufacturers with legitimate products as well as scammers trying to present bogus solutions. As eager as you may be to solve your own hair loss problem, you must be wary. View claims with a jaded eye and consult your physician before you buy.

Descriptions of the products presented in this chapter are primarily based on manufacturers' claims and/or research reports and testimonials published on the Web. Because I have not used these products or formally interviewed anyone who has used them, I cannot personally testify to their effectiveness. However, because they are part of the armamentarium of hair loss products, I feel justified in introducing them briefly. I feel that you should at least know about their availability and that if you are interested in any specific products or approaches, you will gather more information. Please be aware that not one of these products is FDA approved except for minoxidil, which you will note is used in conjunction with certain products. Some products have been manufactured and used in European countries but are not sold in the United States except through Internet sources. I strongly urge you to obtain all the information available before you try any of these products and, by all means, consult your personal physician, dermatologist, or physician hair restoration specialist.

Remember that finasteride is not approved for use in women (See "About Finasteride," chapter 5) and any product that is similar or that incorporates finasteride may not be appropriate for women of child-bearing age.

And lastly, at the rate new hair products are being developed and introduced, by the time this book is in your hands, there will surely be a host of new and exciting products for you to research. As always, I must urge that you please be sure to include your doctor's opinion in your product choices.

CHAPTER 8

FROM THE INSIDE OUT: TAKING CARE OF YOUR SKIN AND HAIR

Protecting your hair, composition of skin, nutritional pathways to healthier skin and hair, essential nutrients, general care of skin, hair and nails

PROTECTING YOUR HAIR, PREVENTING HAIR LOSS

Where do we begin and what can we do specifically to protect our hair and scalp and help prevent hair loss? You've already read at length about the external aspects of hair sickness and hair health. You may have just spent months or even years dealing with hair thinning from androgenetic alopecia or a more complex hair loss problem—some other form of alopecia. Meanwhile, you're asking why there's a *last* chapter on protecting and strengthening hair follicles. Isn't it too late for that? Shouldn't it have come first? Well, of course, creating a healthy head of hair seems to come first, but the whole approach in our society is about externals—what "type" your hair is, dry or oily; shampoos and conditioners to use and not use; volumizers and other products to make your hair appear thicker; moisturizers for hair, those products that make your hair lustrous and shiny; products to protect your hair from the sun—and so on and so on. There's no end to the ways we can treat our hair externally to make it look better. And most of us have grown up thinking that this is all that is necessary. We don't necessarily associate eating carrots or dandelion greens or oats and barley with how our hair grows.

But what we eat and how we think and live can make a difference in the health of our hair and skin, just as it makes a difference in our growth, the functioning of our organ systems, the performance of our reproductive system, the development of diseases of aging, immune system response, preventing illness and, when we need to, recovering from illness. Think about all the possible factors that can lead to hair loss, such as acute illness, surgery, radiation, drug therapies, skin disease, sudden weight loss, high fever, poor blood circulation, diabetes, thyroid disease (hypothyroidism), stress, vitamin and mineral deficiencies, and a poor diet. With this wide range of possible causes, it should be no surprise that maintaining good health status and good nutrition could make a difference in maintaining a healthy scalp and head of hair. So now, in this last chapter, I'm going to lay a foundation for creating healthy hair from the inside out. Even if you've been treated successfully for alopecia, or have found the ideal aesthetic solution, you may want to work on maintaining the healthy follicles you have, or preventing a recurrence or continued hair loss. If you've been diagnosed with alopecia and have found a combination of medical solutions and cosmetic solutions that work for you— I celebrate with you. Whatever your situation, the skin you're in and the hair you have can benefit from following basic nutritional guidelines.

TAKING A LOOK AT THE SKIN WE'RE IN

Healthy hair has to start with healthy skin, because the health of follicles is a skin issue. It only becomes a hair issue when follicles are *not* healthy or, as we've learned, certain body processes have altered due to aging, trauma, or illness.

Let's review the anatomical aspects of skin—what's going on beneath the surface. Understanding the composition of skin will help you understand the importance of nutrients that benefit the skin. Skin is the largest organ in the body and its nutritional status is of greater importance than we generally realize.

First of all, the skin has three layers: the outer *epidermis*, the middle layer or *dermis*, and a fatty layer beneath the first two. The purpose of the paper-thin outer epidermis is actually composed of dead tissue cells that are designed to protect the under layers by holding in moisture and natural oils. The dead cells are constantly sloughed off and replaced by cells that are work-ing their way to the surface to die. Helping our skin to slough off this outer layer is extremely beneficial to the appearance of skin, especially as we age, when the process begins to slow down. Exfoliating scrubs do this job very nicely and help to maintain skin's fresh appearance, whether it's on our face or our bodies. If we don't exfoliate as we age, the natural process will continue to do it for us, but not as efficiently as it did in our youth. The result will be dull, lifeless skin and maybe even allergies and outbreaks that occur because of accumulations of dead cells and debris remaining on the skin. Fortunately, regular shampooing, preferably with mild shampoos, involves massaging the scalp, which helps remove dead skin and debris and doesn't leave all the work to natural exfoliation.

Directly beneath the epidermis, we find basal cells that, in turn, consist of smaller cells called melanocytes that generate melanin. Melanin is the substance that influences your skin color and tone; the melanin you produce is inherited from both of your parents. The dermis layer makes up about 90 percent of your skin and holds the nerves, nerve endings, and blood vessels that carry impulses from the nervous system and circulate blood, nutrients, and oxygen throughout the skin that covers our entire body—and our scalp, of course.

Sweat glands are in this layer as well as the sebaceous glands that are attached to hair follicles and produce oil. When sebaceous glands at the roots of hair follicles are blocked in any way, we're apt to see the development of blackheads and acne, especially in areas where oil production is most active, such as the face, chest, and back. The production of sweat and oil secretions within the dermis creates an acid environment—the acid mantle of the skin—that provides natural protection from infective organisms. Ironically, when we have outbreaks of any kind or wish to prevent them and we use harsh soaps or detergents or soaps that are not pH balanced, we may clear up the outbreak but we're simultaneously destroying the acid mantle of the skin that protects us from infection. What does that say about the value of the antibacterial soaps that are so popular these days? Do we need them? Or should we spend our soap dollars on cleansers that benefit the skin's natural protective mechanism? Oil production by the sebaceous glands will decrease as we age, we can be sure of it. The good part is that skin problems like acne typically clear up; the bad part is that our skin begins to dry, lines begin to form, and we begin to apply oils and moisturizers from the outside. We even use moisturizing shampoos to replenish scalp moisture.

Inside the dermis layer we can also find the substances that give our skin its elasticity and flexibility, things that we don't want to lose but whose production will decline to some degree as we age. Collagen and elastin, for example, are essential to the integrity of skin, but loss is inevitable. Collagen production diminishes at about 1 percent each year starting in our 20 percent, indicating that by the time we're middle aged, collagen production will be about 20 percent less than normal. This varies from person to person and also among skin tones; the darker the skin, the more collagen and elastin to start with, therefore the skin of the average middle-aged dark-skinned woman will not show signs of aging as much as that of a lighter-skinned women. The lines we see forming in our skin as we age are a direct result of the breakdown of elastin and collagen fibers in the dermis and deeper layers of the skin. Young skin with a plentiful supply of elastin and collagen will be resilient, stretching and contracting to maintain its shape. In the absence of sufficient collagen and elastin, skin will droop and develop lines. (I will not say the W word.) Along with the breakdown of collagen and elastin, the skin's natural ability to repair itself also diminishes. The effects of aging combined give us drier skin, less resilient skin, sagging skin, and an inability for the skin itself to keep up with the damage. Keeping up with damage could be particularly important if we're talking about the repair of damaged follicles. As we age, we lose not only the constituents of skin but also certain immune system capabilities that can help restore damage wherever it occurs.

What else damages our skin and scalp? Free radicals, those nasty unstable oxygen molecules riding rampant within our bloodstream and in body tissues, act on our skin as the oxygen in air acts on iron—we begin to oxidize as iron begins to "rust." We produce these free radicals through environmental exposure—that is, when we're exposed to sun, specific toxins such as pesticides, smoke, air pollutants and everyday chemical exposure from cleaning agents, synthetic dyes and perfumes, harsh detergents, certain air fresheners, certain food additives, use of certain types of drugs (they can be either recreational or therapeutic), and even toxic thoughts and emotions (the condition we call stress). The result of free radical production is seen in our metabolic processes, diseases, or conditions that develop as we age, and also in our skin; it becomes dry, stiff, and discolored to some extent and less resilient. Basically, it's not looking healthy any more; it has lost its vitality. We may see this in our skin, hair, or nails as general health declines. But it is not inevitable. There are steps we can take to maintain vitality, reduce damage from free radicals, and ward off many of the effects of aging.

Just from this cursory review of the composition of skin, you can begin to see how the health of skin and hair follicles depends on a process of maintaining a stable internal environment and avoiding or ameliorating an external environment that influences free radical development. It's clear that our approach to protecting our skin and hair follicles, and thereby protecting the health of our hair, is not just from the outside, which has been the focus of this book so far. What we can do to maintain healthy skin and hair by approaching it from the inside is the focus of this chapter.

A BRIEF REVIEW OF HAIR FOLLICLE ACTIVITY

Besides the previous discussion of the composition of skin and what can damage it, you may remember the earlier discussion of the construction of the hair follicle and how it works (see chapter 2). To review briefly, inside each follicle are tiny cells of the matrix involved in synthesizing proteins during the hair growth phase (anagen)—a process that goes on continuously while hair is growing. When the generation of hair stops (telogen), the activity stops. At this time, the hair root is partially dormant and partially destroyed until the follicle resumes its activity. Then a whole new hair root is regenerated and hair production starts all over again. Imagine the energy required to maintain an entire head of hair! The growth cycles of each follicle must build up and tear down the follicle itself, building its product, which is hair, from raw materials—the metabolic constituents that synthesize protein. Ribonucleic acid (RNA) and deoxyribonucleic acid (DNA) must be in abundance in the follicle cells that build protein. Therefore, nutritional building blocks such as folic acid, B^{12}, and other B vitamins must be present in abundance to guarantee that nucleic acid will be present to maintain RNA and DNA in sufficient quantity. Minerals and enzymes must be present to help maintain the biochemical processes and provide the energy to support protein synthesis. Immune system function must be working well to protect against disease or infection. In summary, the essential vitamins, minerals, enzymes, and amino acids must be available to undertake the huge task of maintaining follicle health, protein synthesis, and hair generation—that is, if we want hair growth to continue normally.

NUTRITIONAL PATHWAYS TO HEALTHIER SKIN AND HAIR

I believe that we all want healthy skin and hair, knowing at some level that it's the way we'll look and feel our best. And healthier nails, too, by the way. Whatever we do to nourish our skin and hair will also benefit our nails—they thrive on the same nutrients. The reverse is true, too. If we are not thriving because of illness or deficiencies in basic nutrition, our skin, hair, and nails will reflect this—they will not be looking their best and may give us clues to our general state of health.

Other than maintaining a healthy diet, one that is rich in whole foods and low in the harmful fats and high glycemic foods typically found in manufactured or prepared food products, what can we consume or what supplements can we take to ensure we are maintaining healthy skin, hair, and nails? Part of the answer depends on understanding how nutritional deficiencies may contribute to skin breakdown and to hair loss. The other part of the answer is to understand the function of nutrients noted for their ability to support healthy skin and healthy hair follicles and thereby a healthy scalp (and let's not forget the nails).

Nutrition is a fairly practical matter even though it's happening at a complex cellular level we cannot see and not at a visible level like the nose on our faces and hair on our heads that we see every day. Basically, certain vitamins and minerals are essential to the metabolic pathways that lead to keratin protein metabolism—and keratin protein metabolism is essential to maintaining healthy skin and healthy hair growth. Without these essential vitamins and minerals, the negative environmental effects on the skin will outweigh the positive effects of good external skin care, and changes of some kind will occur in the hair growth process to keep it from continuing normally. Poor nutrition shows in the health of our skin pretty readily. With hair, it's a bit different and it may take longer to notice negative effects. Although the absence of essential vitamins and minerals may not be directly related to hair loss, it is related to impaired hair growth in various ways. The biochemical functions of nutritional factors such as folic acid and vitamin B^{12} are known, for example, to be vital in the synthesis of proteins necessary to skin and hair. Deficiencies of these and other B vitamins interfere with the production of nucleic acids needed for the formation of nucleoproteins within the hair follicle itself. Additionally, high glycogen content has been found in the actively growing cells of hair follicles in the outer root sheath. Glycogen, a carbohydrate found in most body tissues, is understood to be the energy source that supports protein synthesis while hair is in the growth phase, reinforced by the fact that little glycogen is found in follicles during the rest phase. Enzymes that are related to glucose metabolism and the synthesis of glycogen are therefore very important to normal hair growth and must be supplied consistently. Clearly, the minerals and vitamins used by the body as cofactors in protein synthesis must be in sufficient supply within the body to ensure that cell replication within the follicle is maintained and hair growth proceeds normally.

So let's jump from here, where I hope you've begun to see and accept the importance of nutrients in maintaining healthy skin and hair, to outlining some of the nutrients known to nourish the skin, hair, and nails and to provide immune system support.

NUTRIENTS ESSENTIAL TO HEALTHY SKIN, HAIR, AND NAILS

Nutritional assessment is something every physician may do for certain patients to determine whether they are receiving adequate amounts of the nutrients required by the body for optimum health, organ function, and healing when needed. For most patients, this may be a simple question-and-answer session about eating habits, and advice may be given by the physician about reducing or eliminating certain types of foods such as cutting down on saturated fats, reducing sugar intake, or increasing plant sources and decreasing animal sources, depending on each person's health status. If an individual seems to be at risk for malnutrition as a result of illness, or has experienced substantial weight gain or weight loss, the nutritional assessment may be more in depth or the person may be sent to a nutritionist for consultation. A careful evaluation of food intake will be done, including how many meals are eaten each day, who prepares them, what types of foods are consumed, appetite levels, digestive problems—a full range of factors that deal with nutritional intake as well as possible dietary deficiencies. Tests may even be done to evaluate levels of fat, carbohydrates, and protein in the body as well as minerals (e.g., zinc, calcium, and magnesium). The important thing is for the physician to understand the person's ability to obtain, prepare, ingest, digest, metabolize (turn into energy), or absorb nutrients that are essential to body function. Not everyone needs this kind of evaluation, but when we have acute or chronic illness or are not performing as we should, nutritional status is often an indicator of dietary deficiencies that need to be corrected. We can all learn to eat better to maintain our health, manage a chronic disease such as diabetes, or to help us recover from a specific condition. Ask your doctor to refer you to a nutritionist if you think you and your overall health could benefit from nutritional assessment.

Meanwhile, what can we do ourselves to maintain the health of our skin—the body's largest organ—and the hair follicles that produce and maintain our heads of hair? Some of the most notable vitamins and minerals essential to healthy skin, hair, and nails are discussed next along with dietary sources.

- *B vitamins* are known to support the health and growth of scalp hair, partially from its contribution (through B^6, folic acid, and B^{12}) to the formation of hemoglobin, the oxygen-carrying component of red blood cells that distribute oxygen to all body tissues, including the scalp. Healthy hair depends on a constant supply of blood and oxygen and a reduced supply readily results in hair shedding and slow regrowth. Since animal studies have shown that hair loss can occur when B vitamins are lacking, it follows that obtaining a sufficient level of B vitamins, especially including B^3 (niacin), B^5 (pantothenic acid), B^6, biotin, inositol, and folic acid, can benefit hair growth and the maintenance of healthy hair, skin, and nails. Vitamin B^6, for example, is actually a group of three vitamins (pyridoxine, pyridoxal, and pyridoxamine) that are necessary for activation of the enzyme that converts glycogen to glucose and aids in the synthesis and metabolism of protein. Biotin is especially important and deficiencies are shown to result in thinning of hair as well as graying and loss of hair. Biotin is found in peanuts, chocolate, and eggs, it is synthesized naturally in intestinal bacteria, but the synthesized form is not assimilated as well as consumed sources. Reports of a study in which biotin was taken as a supplement showed that the majority of people who participated had improvements in the firmness of their nails and a decrease in brittleness and splitting (Rakel, 2007), a sign that protein metabolism is reflected in the growth and health of nail tissue. We would expect that hair and skin would benefit similarly.

B vitamins can be found readily in foods and are available in supplements such as B complex formulas that contain all the essential B vitamins. Foods high in B vitamins, biotin, and folic acid include peas, beans, lentils, soybeans, brewer's yeast, cauliflower, carrots, nutritional yeast, brown rice, eggs, sunflower seeds, and nuts, among other sources.

- *Vitamin C* (ascorbic acid) deficiencies will result in slower wound healing and gradual degeneration of skin tissue—in fact, its lack will affect all body tissues, including gums and blood vessels. This is largely due to the contribution of vitamin C to the development of collagen, a building block for connective tissue and essential to skin, hair, and nails. When present in sufficient quantities, vitamin C improves blood circulation to body tissues, including the scalp and within the scalp, by improving the integrity of small veins called capillaries. As an antioxidant, vitamin C stimulates the immune system and helps protect body tissues, including skin and the scalp, against infection. It also improves the absorption of iron when supplemental iron is taken to prevent deficiencies or iron deficiency anemia. But primarily vitamin C is needed for the formation of connective tissue that holds our cells together, which is also what makes it vital to tissue repair.

Besides its availability as a supplement, vitamin C can be found in citrus fruits (especially in the white material inside the skins of citrus fruits), cantaloupe, cabbage, and all fresh fruits and vegetables. If we eat enough of a variety of fruits and vegetables, it would be hard for us to become deficient in vitamin C. Remember though that vitamin C is heat labile, which means it is destroyed by heat (also to some extent by sunlight and air). Frozen vegetables lose about 50 percent of their available vitamin C, and frozen fruit about 30 percent. It's best to eat fresh and/or raw fruits and vegetables to get your vitamin C. And don't think you're getting a full dose of vitamin C in hot teas with rose hips; yes, the vitamin is in rose hips, but boiling tea water reduces the amount you can receive.

- *Vitamin E* is found in the body as tocopherols, which are compounds that are naturally occurring antioxidants. Although vitamin E does not seems to be lacking in the average diet and deficiencies are not found, it is known to improve circulation, including circulation to the scalp, which increases the flow of oxygen to scalp tissue, helping to improve the health and growth of hair. As an antioxidant, vitamin E improves immune system protection of the scalp and hair. Avocados, nuts, seeds, and olive oil add vitamin E to the diet.

- *Vitamin A* is called a vitamin although it behaves as a hormone; its active form is retinol. Because it is not synthesized in the body, we must acquire it through external sources. Its primary function is to promote the growth and health of cells and body tissue throughout the body, including the scalp and hair. It accomplishes this by helping to synthesize glycoproteins needed for cell growth, acting almost like a steroid hormone. It is also an antioxidant and free-radical fighter in the body, protecting against infection and cancer. Deficiency of vitamin A can lead to the buildup of cellular debris; if this occurs within hair follicles, it can result in hair loss and dandruff. Vitamin A is primarily found in animal sources, including butter, liver, egg yolks, whole milk, and fish oils, but it is also abundant in nut oils and seeds. Spinach contains some vitamin A, and carrots and other yellow vegetables and fruits (e.g., sweet potato and cantaloupe) contain carotene, a carotenoid that readily converts to vitamin A in the body. Since it doesn't convert at exactly 100 percent, it's best to consume foods high in carotene, like carrots and dark green leafy vegetables. Thyroid-related hair loss can be aided by consuming foods high in vitamin A and iodine (unless you're on a low iodine diet prior to a radioactive iodine scan or treatment for thyroid cancer). Good sources of vitamin A include carrots, spinach, and cold-pressed oils from flaxseeds, walnuts, or pumpkin seeds. Vitamin A can be taken as a supplement but can be toxic in quantities over 10,000 IU daily. Although vitamin A can help ensure adequate nourishment and growth for cells within hair follicles, to complicate matters, excess vitamin A can result in hair loss, so balance must be maintained. Follicular hyperkeratosis, the presence of rough, bumpy skin, can result from vitamin A deficiency.

- *Zinc* is a mineral that stimulates hair growth by boosting the immune system function and by helping to maintain the oil-secreting glands attached to hair follicles. A deficiency of zinc is known to lead to both hair loss and seborrheic dermatitis (dandruff). Good food sources of zinc include fish, eggs, and milk. Whole grains, nuts, seeds, and legumes also contain zinc, but in a form that is not as well assimilated in the body.

- *Silicon*, an essential trace mineral, has been shown to be important to the health of bones and skin, with noticeable effects when ingested or used externally. It aids in the formation of collagen that contributes to the strength and development of skin cells (epithelial cells) and the connective tissue in our bones and joints. In the diet, potatoes, green and red peppers, cucumbers, and bean sprouts are high in silicon.

- *Iron* is a primary constituent of hemoglobin, the iron-bearing protein in red blood cells. Iron deficiency is known to lead to anemia and to

169

hair loss or increased shedding. Although iron sources include animal meats, a nonheme form of iron (the form that does not carry oxygen) is found in plant foods such as spinach, kidney beans, apricots, and raisins. Dietary sources can provide iron that is readily assimilated but in a deficiency, physicians may prescribe supplemental sources along with vitamin C to help absorption.

A DIET THAT CONTRIBUTES TO HEALTHY SKIN AND ENCOURAGES HAIR GROWTH

We cannot say definitively that a specific diet will make hair grow in the presence of balding, either due to genetic reasons or caused by a specific underlying condition. However, maintaining a healthy head of hair certainly requires overall good nutrition, just as any other body process benefits from good nutrition. A diet rich in silica, calcium, and iron is believed to help reduce hair loss or, depending on the individual's genetic makeup, prevent hair loss (Chaney, 2002). Minerals can be added to the diet by consuming sea vegetables like seaweed and green leafy vegetables like kale, spinach, chard, and collards. Silica is found in raw oats as in muesli or granola. Dried fruits, especially apricots, provide a good source of iron.

Our objectives in eating a certain way to have healthier skin and hair are to nourish the skin, to support essential body processes and follicular hair generation, and to maintain a healthy immune status so we can fight infection effectively. For example, we learned earlier in chapter 2 that hair is composed primarily of proteins. A diet rich in protein is easy enough to obtain, whether you are a meat eater or a vegetarian, and it's essential to maintaining the health of your hair. For optimum overall health and to achieve our specific objectives for healthy skin, hair, and nails, we need to follow a food plan based on consuming whole foods rather than prepared or manufactured foods—in that way, we get our nutrients without processing, without alteration, and without damaging saturated or hydrogenated fats or the high-glycemic-index foods that raise our sugar levels (glucose levels) to undesirable heights without contributing to our nutrition. These fats and sugars are the so-called empty calories that only add pleasure while we eat them and add extra pounds while we're not watching.

A healthy whole-foods diet includes whole grains (brown rice, millet, buckwheat, spelt, and quinoa) and wholegrain products (cereals, pastas, crackers, and breads, among others), fresh fruits and vegetables, and quality protein sources such as beans, peas, legumes, nuts, seeds, fish and poultry, lean meats in moderation, eggs, and low-fat dairy. Things to avoid or reduce include animal fats, hydrogenated or trans fats, and oils that have been extracted at high temperatures. Cold-pressed oils such as canola and olive oil are best for us for routine use. Processed sweets and baked goods should also be reduced or avoided and, if you have diabetes or are watching your weight, it's best to consume only minimal amounts of foods high on the glycemic index. Some of the foods high on the comprehensive glycemic index list are white bread, white rice, potatoes, bananas, glucose (pure sugar), and honey (find the glycemic index at www.drweil.com or Google it).

You can also find the Food Guide Pyramid, a graphic representation of recommendations by the U.S. Department of Agriculture (USDA) for a balanced diet, depicted on certain food packaging and shown on the USDA Web site (see Resources). The pyramid shows the ideal percentages we should eat of various types of food we consume regularly. Rather than being based on acquiring certain nutrients, it's based on achieving a balance of quality protein, fats, and carbohydrates. You cannot go wrong if you follow it, but you'll note that it does not specify what *not* to eat, including refined foods such as white flour, white sugar, and refined or prepared foods of any kind that may fill your tummy but lack nutrients. The process of refining and prepackaging foods often removes essential nutrients, so manufacturers and their food chemists try to add them back ("fortified with …") to create an "enriched" product. But your body does know the difference between whole foods and chemical constituents and may not thrive on these nutrient-depleted foods, whereas whole foods consumed without processing will give you the highest percentage of the nutrients they contain naturally.

Regardless of what principles guide your food choices—a whole-foods diet or the food pyramid—remember that it's 90 percent of your diet that will determine your health status; you can afford to play a little with the remaining 10 percent just so you don't feel overly restricted. (Restriction isn't always good for us, either.) Every one of us goes to a restaurant or a wedding feast once in a while and we splurge a little without losing our health.

DELAYING AGING TO DELAY AGE-RELATED HAIR LOSS

Controversial, yes, but worth exploring on an individual basis, the idea of starting early to reduce the characteristics of aging is not going to prevent hair loss if we're genetically susceptible, but it is believed to delay the inevitable hair loss or thinning associated with androgenetic alopecia. This complementary medicine approach to hair loss may be the long route, but many holistic practitioners recommend that it's a sure route to reducing the acceleration of aging, thereby reducing the onset of age-related disease and deterioration in the health of our skin and hair. We know that both skin and hair can reveal the effects of changing body processes, hormones, and metabolism. The theory is that humans cannot entirely avoid these changes, but can slow them, staying younger longer. Is there someone who doesn't want that?

A well-balanced whole-foods diet with essential nutrients is the place to start. Again—nutritionists and practitioners of integrative medicine advise it strongly—avoid eating processed and refined foods, particularly white flour, white sugar, carbonated soft drinks, hydrogenated oils, food additives, and prepared foods—the frozen dinners, fast foods, and overly processed nutrient-depleted foods that are manufactured to make life "easier" for busy people. Eating a whole-foods diet gives us a ready source of the nutrients we need for health and supply the energy for our active lives. What could be easier than eating food as nature has given it to us? A basic whole-foods diet includes whole grains; a range of green, yellow, and red vegetables; high-quality protein; and oils derived from cold-pressed olives, nuts, and seeds. Protein sources include fish, poultry, and lean meats; eggs; and a moderate amount of dairy products such as milk and cheese. Eat your sweets as whole fruits, knowing that the occasional slice of wedding cake or cookie will not hurt, but sugar itself (e.g., white sugar, brown sugar, molasses, and high-fructose corn syrup) should be avoided as much as possible in the daily diet. Lots of whole-food sweeteners are available, including agave syrup, barley malt, and brown rice syrup. It's easy to switch and you'll feel better without the sugar highs.

Superfoods have also been identified as anti-aging or longevity foods, but all superfoods are from whole-food sources such as greens and whole grains. It's easy to add superfoods to the diet through supergreens (chlorella, spirulina, micro-algae extracts) and sprouts as a ready source of high-quality protein. Fresh leafy greens and the colorful berries (organic only, because these small fruits absorb pesticides so readily), such as blueberries, raspberries, strawberries, and blackberries, can be eaten in season.

VITAMIN PRODUCTS MARKETED FOR HAIR GROWTH

Since vitamins, proteins, and minerals have long been considered to be necessary for healthy hair, skin, and nails, various preparations are promoted as being of special benefit for healthy follicles and hair growth. To make it easier for you to get the nutrients you need for healthy hair, skin, and nails, nutritional supplements are being combined in formulations sold for this specific purpose. One example among many is the extra-strength vitamin preparation called Viviscal for Women, which has been called the "miracle mane" by *Cosmopolitan* magazine. It is prepared in tablet form and is considered by some to be the essential hair vitamin. Viviscal was developed in Finland and is manufactured by a Finnish company. Its primary ingredients include vitamin C, cartilaginous marine extract, acerola extract, and silica compounds. The "cartilaginous marine extract" may be shark or other marine animal cartilage that provides a rich source of amino acid proteins. Acerola is a botanical that grows in tropical climates; it has a cherrylike fruit noted for its high vitamin C content. Testimonials and scientific studies are available to support Viviscal's results (www.onlyhairloss.com/viviscal_tablets.htm). Other options include purchasing supplements separately or in mixed vitamin formulations, or consuming foods known to contain the vitamins and minerals you feel will boost the health of your skin and hair. Whole-foods markets usually have a comprehensive selection of vitamin, mineral, and herbal supplements, and the department is often divided according to health-related categories, making it easy to find supplements that work for specific needs. Clerks assigned to the department are sometimes very knowledgeable, but it's helpful to have your researched list with you so you go home with the nutrients you need.

A FINAL WORD ABOUT YOUR HEALTH AND THE HEALTH OF YOUR SCALP AND HAIR

This is not a book on nutrition. There is so much more to learn about total body nutrition than I can possibly discuss here; I have merely scratched the surface. What I hope the discussion in this chapter has done, however, is to inspire your interest in cultivating healthy skin, hair, and nails from the inside out, not just finding external solutions for your hair loss problem. If you have a form of alopecia that has troubled you, please be assured that you are still a whole, beautiful being with a full range of options available to you for treating your condition externally and internally.

Please look over the Resources section at the back of the book; the Web sites, organizations, and books are resources that can add to your knowledge of your condition and your treatment options, and help you with your choice of procedures and products. The organizational listings include resources that can help you find a physician hair replacement specialist near you. These resources will also remind you of the many options open to you and help you decide what might be worth exploring. There is a solution that's perfect for you. Follow your instincts and get the information and assistance you need to help you handle your alopecia and your health.

Be well. Be happy.

BIBLIOGRAPHY

Balch, P. A. *Prescription for Nutritional Healing: The A to Z Guide to Supplements*. New York: Penguin Putnam, 2002.

Bernstein, R. M. "Hair Transplantation.: Center for Hair Restoration, 2008. http://www.bernsteinmedical.com. March 15, 2008.

————. "Hair Cloning and Genetic Engineering." Center for Hair Restoration, 2008. http://www.bernsteinmedical.com. March 9, 2008.

Chaney, S. G. "Principles of Nutrition I: Macronutrients," in *Textbook of Biochemistry with Clinical Correlations*. T. M Devlin, ed. New York: Wiley-Liss, 2002.

————. "Principles of Nutrition II: Micronutrients," in *Textbook of Biochemistry with Clinical Correlations*. T. M. Devlin, ed. New York: Wiley-Liss, 2002.

Chapman, Lynne, ed. "The New Look of Wigs–Cranial Hair Prosthesis." Bella Online: The Voice of Women, 2008. http://www.bellaonline.com/articles/art5574.asp. August 2, 2008.

Chartier, M. B., D. M. Hoss, and J. M. Grant-Kels. "Approach to the Adult Female Patient with Diffuse Nonscarring Alopecia," *Journal of the American Academy of Dermatology* 47 (2002): 809–18.

Cummings, C. W., ed. "Pathophysiology: Forms and Etiologies of Alopecia," in *Otolaryngology: Head & Neck Surgery*, 4th ed. Philadelphia: Mosby, 2005.

————. "Surgical Management," in *Otolaryngology: Head & Neck Surgery*, 4th ed. Philadelphia: Mosby, 2005.

Eickhorst, K. M. and E. Levit. "Diseases of the Hair," in *Conn's Current Therapy 2007*, 59th ed. R. E. Rakel, ed. Philadelphia: Saunders Elsevier, 2007.

Goyal, S., and R. A. Schwartz. "Loose Anagen Syndrome," *The Medscape Journal* (October 19, 2006). http://www.emedicine.com/derm/topic768.htm. May 23, 2008.

Habif, T. "Alopecia Areata," in *Clinical Dermatology*, 4th ed. New York: Mosby, 2004.

Hadshiew, I. N., K. Foitzik, P. C. Arck, and R. Paus. "Burden of Hair Loss: Stress and the Underestimated Psychosocial Impact of Telogen Effluvium and Androgenetic Alopecia," *Journal of Investigative Dermatology* 123 (2004): 445–57.

"Hair Loss, Baldness, Diet/Food Therapy/Nutrition/Vitamins." Holistic online. 2007. ICBS. http://www.holisticonline.com/remedies/hair/hair_loss-nutrition.htm. February 28, 2008.

"Hair Loss & Restoration in Women." International Society of Hair Restoration Surgery. http://www.ishrs.org/articles/hair-loss-women.htm. May 21, 2008.

Harper, J. C. "Antiandrogen Therapy for Skin and Hair Disease," *Dermatologic Clinics* 24 (2006): 2.

Hennessey, J., and L. Wartofsky. "Hashimoto's Disease," *Journal of Clinical Endocrinology and Metabolism* 92 (2007): 7.

Mayo Clinic. "Trichotillomania (Hair-Pulling Disorder). Mayo Foundation for Medical Education and Research (January 25, 2007). http://www.mayoclinic.com/print/ trichotillomania/DS00895/METHOD=print&DS. March 30, 2008.

Norris, D. A. "Alopecia Areata: Current State of Knowledge," *Journal of the American Academy of Dermatology* 51 (2004): 1.

Northrup, Christiane, MD. *The Wisdom of Menopause*. New York: Bantam, 2001.

Norwood, O. T. "Incidence of Female Androgenetic Alopecia (Female Pattern Alopecia)," *Dermatologic Surgery* 27 (2001): 1.

Olsen, E. A. "Iron Deficiency and Hair Loss: The Jury is Still Out," *Journal of the American Academy of Dermatology* 54 (2006): 5.

Otberg, N., A. M. Finner, and J. Shapiro. "Androgenetic Alopecia," *Endocrinology and Metabolism Clinics* 36 (2007): 2.

Rakel, R. E., ed. "Nutritional Assessment: Summary of Major Nutrients," in *Textbook of Family Medicine*, 7th ed. Philadelphia: Saunders, 2007.

Roberts, J., P. Rich, and F. Parker. "Disorders of Hair, Nails, and Pigmentation," in *Textbook of Primary Care Medicine*, 3rd ed. John Noble, ed. St. Louis: Mosby, 2001.

Ross-Flanigan, N. "Antimalarial Drugs." Gale Encyclopedia of Medicine. www.healthatoz.com. May 7, 2008.

Schwartz, R. A., and B. D. Seiff. "Anagen Effluvium," *The Medscape Journal* (May 30, 2207). http://www.emedicine.com/derm/topic894.htm. April 3, 2008.

Smith, N., and A. Welch, eds. "Through Thick and Thin," *Vogue Magazine* (April 2008).

Sperling, S. "Resources for Women." Hair Club. http://www.hairclub.com. August 3, 2008.

Springer, K., M. Brown, and D. L. Stulberg. "Common Hair Loss Disorders," *American Family Physician* 68 (2003): 93–102.

Stough, D. "Female Hair Loss." The Hair Loss Learning Center. http://www .hairlosslearningcenter.org/content/hair-loss-research. February 28, 2008.

Stoppler, M. C. "Stress Management." Medicine Net (April 10, 2008). http://www.medicinet.com. W. C. Shiel, ed. August 10, 2008.

Tessmer, K. A. "Diet and Hair Loss." http://www.stophairlossnow.co.uk. August 12, 2008.

Thiedke, C. C. "Alopecia in Women," *American Family Physician* 67 (2003): 5.

Tosti, A., and M. Pazzaglia. "Drug Reactions Affecting Hair: Diagnosis," *Dermatologic Clinics* 25 (2007): 2.

Trost, L. B., W. F. Bergfeld, and E. Calogeras. "The Diagnosis and Treatment of Iron Deficiency and Its Potential Relationship to Hair Loss," *Journal of the American Academy of Dermatology* 54 (2006): 5.

"Types of Hair Loss." American Hair Loss Association (2007). http:// www.americanhairloss.org/women_hair_loss/introduction.asp. March 20, 2008.

U.S. Department of Agriculture. *The Food Guide Pyramid*. Hayesville, MD: Human Nutrition Information Service, 1992.

Venning, V. A. and R. P. R. Dawber. "Patterned Androgenetic Alopecia in Women." *Journal of the American Academy of Dermatology* 18 (1988): 1073–77.

Whiting, D. A. "Chronic Telogen Effluvium: Increased Scalp Hair Shedding in Middle-Aged Women," *Journal of the American Academy of Dermatology* 35 (1996): 899–906.

Wolever, T. M., D. J. Jenkins, A. L. Jenkins, and R. G. Josse. "The Glycemic Index Methodology and Clinical Implications," *American Journal of Clinical Nutrition* 54 (1991): 846.

RESOURCES

Web Sites

Center for Hair Restoration. Dr. Robert M. Bernstein, MD
www.bersteinmedical.com

Cicatricial Alopecia Research Foundation (CARF)
www.carfintl.org

The Hair Loss Directory
www.hairlossdirect.com

Hair Loss Talk
www.hairlosstalk.com/newsletter

Hair Restoration Network
www.hairrestorationnetwork.com

Hair Transplant Network
www.hairtransplantnetwork.com

The Bald Truth (support group, radio program, Web site)
www.thebaldtruth.com

Trichotillomania Learning Center, Inc.
www.trich.org

Types of Hair Loss (a comprehensive review of all types of alopecia by
the American Hair Loss Association)
www.americanhairloss.org/types-of-hair-loss/introduction.asp

Organizations

American Hair Loss Association
www.membership@americanhairloss.org

American Hair Loss Council
www.ahlc.org

American Society of Dermatology
www.asd.org

Coalition of Independent Hair Restoration Physicians
www.hairlosstalk.org/content/restoration-physicians/our-physicians.asp

International Alliance of Hair Restoration Surgeons (IAHRS)
www.iahrs.org

International Society of Hair Restoration Surgery (ISHRS)
1-800-444-2737
info@ishrs.org

National Alopecia Areata Foundation (NAAF)
www.naaf.org

INDEX

NORTH COUNTRY LIBRARY SYSTEM

0 11 01 0339805 0

APR - - 2012